Health$_2$O

Tap into the Healing Powers of Water to
Fight Disease, Look Younger, and Feel Your Best

· · ·

Alexa Fleckenstein, M.D.
with Roanne Weisman

New York Chicago San Francisco Lisbon London Madrid Mexico City
Milan New Delhi San Juan Seoul Singapore Sydney Toronto

Library of Congress Cataloging-in-Publication Data

Fleckenstein, Alexa.
    Health₂O / Alexa Fleckenstein, with Roanne Weisman.
        p.   cm.
    ISBN-13: 978-0-07-147499-3 (alk. paper)
    ISBN-10: 0-07-147499-4
    1. Hydrotherapy.   2. Water Therapeutic use.   3. Water—Health
aspects.   I. Weisman, Roanne, 1952–   II. Title.

    RM252.F54   2007
    613.2'87—dc22   2006038286

1 2 3 4 5 6 7 8 9 10 11 12 13 14 15   FGR/FGR   0 9 8 7

ISBN-13: 978-0-07-147499-3
ISBN-10:   0-07-147499-4

McGraw-Hill books are available at special quantity discounts to use as premiums and sales promotions, or for use in corporate training programs. For more information, please write to the Director of Special Sales, Professional Publishing, McGraw-Hill, Two Penn Plaza, New York, NY 10121-2298. Or contact your local bookstore.

The information contained in this book is intended to provide helpful and informative material on the subject addressed. It is not intended to serve as a replacement for professional medical advice. A health care professional should be consulted regarding your specific situation.

This book is printed on acid-free paper.

With love and Danke schön to my husband, Rudolf Jaenisch, and to Dorothée, Johan, and Emily

—A.F.

To my husband and best friend, Michael, and to our children, Benjamin and Elizabeth, with deep love and gratitude

—R.W.

CONTENTS

Introduction   ix

PART **I**   WATER:
              OUR WELLSPRING

CHAPTER 1   THE HEALING PROPERTIES
              OF WATER   3

CHAPTER 2   CREATING BALANCE:
              HOW WATER THERAPY WORKS   7

CHAPTER 3   TRANSFORMING YOUR BATHROOM
              INTO A HEALING WATER SPA   17

CHAPTER 4   IN THE SHOWER   23

CHAPTER 5   IN THE BATHTUB   29

CHAPTER 6   AT THE SINK   41

CHAPTER 7   OUTSIDE THE HOME   47

CHAPTER 8 WATER TREATMENTS FOR SELECTED HEALTH ISSUES 55

PART 2 MOVEMENT:
TO REST IS TO RUST

CHAPTER 9 GETTING STARTED:
THE TWO-MINUTE EXERCISE REVOLUTION 73

CHAPTER 10 STAYING MOTIVATED TO MOVE 77

CHAPTER 11 GO WITH THE FLOW:
EXERCISE FOR THE LAZY 87

CHAPTER 12 PERFECT POSTURE:
MOVING WITH THE FLOW OF WATER 99

CHAPTER 13 BREATHING:
YOUR MOST IMPORTANT MOVEMENT 107

PART 3 FRESH FOOD:
BURSTING WITH WATER AND FLAVOR,
GIVING LIFE

CHAPTER 14 HEALTH-BY-WATER NUTRITION:
FRESHNESS IS EVERYTHING! 115

CHAPTER 15 THE JOY OF EATING:
MAKING LIFE-AFFIRMING CHOICES 129

CHAPTER 16 WEIGHT LOSS:
NEVER DIET AGAIN 139

PART 4 HERBS:
VITAL GREENS, LIQUID MEDICINE

CHAPTER 17 CHOOSING AND BUYING
HERBAL PRODUCTS 165

CHAPTER 18 HEALING HERBS AND SPICES
IN THE KITCHEN 175

PART 5 LIFE BALANCE:
FOLLOWING NATURE'S RHYTHMS

CHAPTER 19 THE TIDES WITHIN US 189

CHAPTER 20 RESTORING LIFE BALANCE TO HEAL
COMMON HEALTH PROBLEMS 195

CHAPTER 21 PUTTING IT ALL TOGETHER:
THE FIVE WATER ESSENTIALS IN ACTION 201

A Final Word: Conserving the Earth's Water 205
Selected References 209
Index 213

INTRODUCTION

I n the fall of 1849, a young seminary student in Dillingen, Bavaria, was dying. The once sturdy young man had become emaciated. A cough rattled him. Every night his sheets were drenched in sweat. In the morning, he often found blood on his pillow.

The student was Sebastian Kneipp, a poor weaver's son from a small Bavarian village. The change from his village to the crowded, unhealthy conditions in the dormitory and seminary took a tremendous toll on his health. The lack of fresh air, fresh food, and exercise brought about consumption (tuberculosis) in the once strapping young man. Tuberculosis was rampant and incurable in the nineteenth century.

When his physicians had given up on him and he was near death, Sebastian Kneipp desperately searched the seminary library for a cure for consumption. By chance, he unearthed an old tract describing a cold-water cure. Having nothing to lose, he followed the advice of the booklet and jumped into the chilly waters of the Danube River three times a week. He dressed without toweling off (he did not own a towel) and walked home to bed. This barbaric treatment cured him, astonishing his fellow students, teachers, and doctors. He later went on to develop a complete system of health, which he called the Five Pillars of

Health. This nature-based system swept Europe and the world. The *Washington Post* called Sebastian Kneipp one of the three most influential men in the world at that time. (The other two men were President William McKinley and Prince Otto von Bismarck.)

Nowadays, I would not forgo modern medications for treating tuberculosis—although, with drug-resistant strains on the rise, we might have to rethink our approach. But for many other diseases, Sebastian Kneipp's water cure is needed now more than ever because it summons the innate healing powers of our bodies. For my patients, I have adjusted his system to the twenty-first century and busy American life. But the system is still based on the life-giving properties of water, using what I call the Five Water Essentials:

1. **Water:** Life came from the ocean, and today our cells still carry the sea within. Water makes up about 70 percent of our bodies and is far from being an unimportant filler. Because of our ocean past, water inside and outside our bodies heals and rejuvenates.
2. **Movement:** A moving river cleans itself. But stagnant waters rot. To keep our cells functioning, we have to move the water inside our bodies—using and defying gravity—and become supple and fluid as flowing river waters.
3. **Nutrition:** Foodstuffs are the building blocks of our bodies. Plants assimilate light and drink water. Only when fresh (not artificially processed) are they nourishing victuals. Bursting with moisture, such plants—and animals fed on them—will build healthy bodies and supply our cells with life-giving energy.
4. **Herbs:** Water pulls minerals from the soil into every plant cell, and we can harvest this healing power: in herbal medicines as teas and infusions, and in the kitchen with tasty herbs and spices.

5. **Life balance:** When we follow the rhythms of the natural ebb and flow of life, our bodies and minds can relax, rejuvenate, and heal.

Incorporating water and the water-based essentials of natural health into our daily lives is as effortless, fast, and inexpensive as the water that comes out of your faucet when you turn it on. It's effortless because water works naturally with our ancient biology, fast because these health-promoting measures take only minutes to include in your life, and inexpensive because the Five Water Essentials use only what the earth provides.

Why You Need the Five Water Essentials

Biologically we are still very much like our cave-dwelling ancestors. Over millions of years, our bodies have been exposed to the elements: cold, rain, sun, wind. Constant changes challenged our systems to adapt. There were no air-conditioned rooms in the summer or central heating in the winter. Now our bodies are barely exposed to the weather outside, and we have become alienated from the natural elements.

Cold and hunger made cave dwellers roam the fields; food had to be gathered, plucked, collected, trapped, hunted, preserved, and stored. For this active life our bodies were made for movement—not for just opening the refrigerator when we're hungry. The rewards of civilization may be comfortable, but they can also ruin our health. On the one hand, we are overstressed from trying to do it all in the modern world. On the other, too little is asked from us. We are not exposed to dirt anymore, so our immune systems cannot learn how to fight infections. Since we can just pop in a car and go wherever we want without really moving, our muscles wither and cannot heat up our body, make our blood circulate, and eliminate toxins.

The Five Water Essentials Work Naturally with Our Bodies

Our biology still operates exactly as it did in ancient times, when our immune systems were stimulated by the effects of living outdoors, where we were in constant motion in the search for food and shelter. We have evolved over millions of years, and one century of electricity, central heating, and automation is not long enough to cause significant changes in our biology. Many of the illnesses of modern life, including diabetes, heart disease, autoimmune disorders, depression, chronic pain, obesity, and cancer, are the responses of an immune system that no longer functions as it should. We can, however, improve our health by making a few simple modifications to our lifestyles. One of the most important modifications is embracing the power of water.

Water treatments restore some of our evolutionary birthright. Because we are still in the Stone Age biologically, we will be healthier the more we can emulate and reinstitute the cave people's surroundings. Of course, we do not want to return to the cave. But research has found that cold water, applied at least once a day to the body, restores some of the body's ancient functions and balances some of the damaging effects of modern life. For example, in a pilot study of the immune effects from water therapy with a small number of breast cancer patients, researchers found significantly increased numbers of disease-fighting cells in every category examined, including neutrophils, monocytes, and lymphocytes. And a study of 68 patients with high cholesterol in London's Thrombosis Research Institute reported a highly significant reduction in both total and LDL ("bad") cholesterol, along with other benefits, after three months of cold-water therapy. This study (like many other similar ones) actually used cold water *immersion*—not what I recommend in this book. But they all show that cold water has a powerful effect on the body. Cold water does not just pearl off from the skin: it drives profound internal changes.

Reaping the Benefits of the Five Water Essentials

You do not need a spa and a trained person to experience the healing power of the Five Water Essentials. Basically, all you need is a water source—a sink, a bathtub, or even a beach or a creek would suffice—and a few simple instructions on how to move, eat, and live according to the flow of water and the flow of nature. This book will show you how to take advantage of all that the Five Water Essentials have to offer, from general wellness to healing of specific conditions, to weight loss, all by following simple, basic tips.

This book is divided into five parts, each one representing one element of the Five Water Essentials. Part 1 of this book explains why water therapy works and how you can easily use it at home to improve your health and invigorate your body, mind, and spirit. One special feature of this section is a chapter on how to transform your bathroom into your own personal healing water spa. You'll also be provided with step-by-step instructions for treating specific health conditions by using a variety of simple water techniques.

Part 2 focuses on the importance of movement and shows you that just as a river needs to be moving in order to remain clean and toxin free, so, too, does your body and every cell within it. This section of the book offers easy exercises to keep you moving, including two-minute exercises that will help turn your health around, as well as exercises for the "lazy" that will motivate you to go with the flow and reap the benefits of simple but powerful movements.

Part 3 focuses on the third element of the Five Water Essentials: fresh, natural foods. This section gives health-by-water tips for eating healthier and more consciously. They will help you fight disease and melt away pounds by eating fresh, organic foods that are close to nature.

Part 4 will provide you with all you need to know about herbs—what they are, how to buy them, and how they heal. Many herbs are used for medicinal purposes, and in this section, you'll find out how to use them. Water pulls essential nutrients from the soil into the cells of herbs, making herbs and spices so critical to your health and well-being.

Part 5 puts it all together by explaining the importance of overall balance, harmony, and natural order in your life. You'll be shown how to put all of the elements of the Five Water Essentials into action in a sample day, and you'll be reminded of the importance of balancing work and play, activity and sleep. The natural ebb and flow rhythms in the ocean give you a model for balance and harmony that are the keys to creating a peaceful and healthy life.

In the Final Word, an old tale and a new story remind us again of our most precious commodity, water, and how to preserve it.

Let's plunge in now and discover the first element of the Five Water Essentials: water, our wellspring!

PART I

WATER

OUR WELLSPRING

While I trained in European Natural Medicine, I stayed at a spa hotel in Bavaria, in Bad Wörishofen—the tiny town where Sebastian Kneipp practiced his water cure. At five o'clock in the morning, I was awakened by the sound of somebody turning a key in the lock. I opened my eyes to pitch-black darkness. A female bath master holding a bucket of very cold water switched on the light (and now I remembered that she was part of the package deal). She ordered me out of bed. So there I was standing on the rug, half asleep, in the middle of the night—stark naked and apprehensive of what would come. With a wet cloth, the sturdy woman, who decidedly looked not amused, washed me down quickly, from top to bottom. Vividly I remember her mopping round and round on my belly with her washcloth—ice-cold it felt. With a curt nod, she gathered her things, ordered me back into bed, switched off the light, and was gone. It was a weird feeling, returning to my sleep-warm eiderdowns wet. For a moment I worried about the eiderdowns and the bedcovers and the rug, and then I just fell asleep again, blissfully warm and snug.

CHAPTER 1

THE HEALING PROPERTIES OF WATER

I magine a substance that is free, is available to all, and has remarkable powers to keep you young and healthy. It boosts the disease-fighting cells of your immune system, reduces chronic pain, improves your breathing and digestion, normalizes your blood pressure, improves your skin tone, and lifts your mood. The substance, of course, is water.

Why does water have this healing power for humans? Life came out of the ocean, and to this day, the primal ocean is still circulating in us. Each of our cells today has exactly the same salinity (0.9 percent) as when for the first time a membrane grew around some seawater with nucleic acids and formed a cell.

More than four million years ago, our forebears left the oceans and eventually evolved into what we are today: upright humans. But we can never venture far from water. Water is the most abundant chemical on earth, but clean water is getting scarcer even in developed countries. The United Nations declared a Decade of Water in 2005 to address the worldwide problem of shortage and pollution of water.

The UN Decade of Water may have just begun, but humans have always known the value of water. The Greeks, for example, laid the foundation for modern science by speculating about the nature of matter. Thales postulated that water was the fundamental element of everything, because only water could be found in all three states: solid, fluid, and gaseous. Throughout human history, water has been used in holy rituals of many world religions. Water is sacred because it renews us. The water molecule shaped our environments and our history; it shapes our bodies every day, and it will shape our future.

How Water Helps Your Body Function

Water makes up about 70 percent of the human body and about 20 to 90 percent of animal and plant tissue. Water is so useful because it is a superior solvent, allowing dissolved substances (especially minerals) to be transported throughout the body. In addition, water's magnetic and electrical powers are critically important for cell function.

Without food, we can survive a few weeks—without water, only a few days. Only water can bless us with inside and outside renewal. Not only does it make us feel better, it can also make us *look* better. The body needs water in every cell to accomplish all of its important metabolic and hormonal functions.

The Functions of Water Inside Your Body

On the inside of your body, water serves many crucial purposes:

- Filling cells with fluid so that your tissues are firm and not limp
- Transporting molecules from outside to inside your body (digestion), thus nourishing your body
- Eliminating toxins from your body
- Making blood circulation possible
- Maintaining the pH (acidity/alkalinity) balance in the body
- Lubricating joints and cushioning intervertebral discs
- Enabling chemical and enzymatic reactions inside the body
- Regulating body temperature and many other functions, thus promoting balance, harmony, and health

To bathe every one of your gazillions of cells in this wonderful fluid, you have to drink the right amount of water every day. Too much water dilutes precious bodily substances such as electrolytes, salts, and minerals; your urine will look colorless. Too little water impedes your kidneys' ability to flush out waste products; your urine will look dark. What is enough? A rough estimate of the right amount is seven cups of water per day for a person of average height and weight. With heat and exercise, you'll need more. Your urine should be light yellow when you achieve the optimal balance.

The Functions of Water on the Inside and Outside of Your Body

More than a hundred years of science and research have demonstrated that cold water splashed on the body is an effective healing agent. As Sebastian Kneipp discovered, cold water stimulates the body's ability to heal itself. Cold water can do more than just wash away sweat, dirt, old skin cells, bacteria, and viruses:

What a Cold Shower Can Do for You
- Enhance immunity against infections and cancer
- Give your glands (thyroid, adrenals, ovaries/testes) a boost, improving hormonal activity
- Jump-start your mood and motivation
- Crank up your metabolism to fight type 2 diabetes, obesity, gout, rheumatic diseases, depression, and more
- Normalize your blood pressure
- Decrease chronic pain
- Train and improve your blood circulation
- Detoxify your body
- Fight fatigue
- Strengthen exhausted, irritable nerves
- Rejuvenate, heal, and tone the skin
- Deepen your breathing

- Help with insomnia
- Improve kidney function
- Reduce swelling and edema
- Improve lymphatic circulation, thereby increasing immune function
- Reduce stress by regulating your autonomic nervous system
- Regulate temperature, fighting chronically cold hands and cold feet and excessive sweating
- Keep your hair healthy
- Improve hemorrhoids and varicose veins
- Reduce aches and pains

With these wonderful benefits of water, you might be eager to start your cold shower immediately. But don't simply believe my list. Imagine what an amazing thing I am claiming here: water hits your skin, pearls off—and still effects changes deep inside your body! Before you hop under the cold stream, learn from the next chapter how water works these wonders in your body.

CHAPTER 2

CREATING BALANCE
HOW WATER THERAPY WORKS

Water can smooth stones and create canyons. So think what it can do for your body when applied day after day. Water on your skin stimulates the nerve endings just under the skin and sets off chain reactions inside your body. Never underestimate the power of water! Just a few seconds of water on your body every day has a powerful impact on your health.

Maintaining Balance

The human body has many self-regulating mechanisms that maintain the ideal balance, or homeostasis. These mechanisms include temperature adaptation, glands and their hormones, the immune system, the pressure exerted by the heart and the blood vessels, the excitation of the nervous system including the brain, the metabolic and electrolyte mechanisms, the activities of intake and elimination, the circadian rhythm (the natural cycle of waking and sleeping), the working of the muscles through movements, the "breathing" via the skin, the oxygen uptake and carbon dioxide elimination, and scores more. All of them are linked and interconnected and forever need to be adjusted to a new balance. Your body knows best its own healthy middle ground—and can maintain good health provided that not too many undue stresses are straining your system.

Water therapy—especially cold-water therapy—helps your body achieve this balance.

Balancing with Cold Water

A cold shower will lower high blood pressure and raise low blood pressure. How can one single procedure be beneficial for two conditions that are diametrically opposed? The secret is that cold-water therapy helps the body to normalize, to return to its inborn balance.

Disease can be described as an imbalance in the body—blood pressure that is too high or too low, too much fat, too little energy, too much heat, too little blood, too much blood, too much potassium, too little calcium, and so on. (Certainly, some diseases do not fall into these categories, but they are rare.) Natural treatments like water therapy stimulate the body to use its own order-creating systems to regulate itself to a middle ground. Each living being, plant or animal, has been designed by nature to come to a point of internal balance, where everything is in equilibrium. This balancing goes on constantly. A myriad of biochemical processes fine-tunes your body's functioning in split-second time. Cold water can be a powerful tool to entice the bodily systems to get back to normal.

How Cold Water Balances Your System

On a molecular level, when cold water stimulates your skin, certain substances are produced and secreted in cells in and under your skin. These substances, in turn, stimulate certain other cells in your body to secrete other substances, and so on. A cascade of active and powerful molecules is created just by a few seconds of cold water on your skin. All these molecules float around in your body, sometimes destined to go to a distant site, but more often only for a few nanoseconds before they hit their nearby targets and are rendered inactive again by other small molecules.

Research has shown that those small molecules integrate the body's neurological (brain and nerves) and endocrine (glands and hormones) functions and the immune (defense) system. Together, they create a super system, which we now call the neuro-immuno-endocrine system. Sometimes it is also called psycho-neuro-immune system. Whatever its name, you can be sure that your body has in place a network, which can function optimally only if served optimally. And as we have seen, people who are fast-forwarded into the electronic age lack many of the stimuli of the natural environment that held the network in balance for millions of years. Cold water on your skin helps to bring this complex network of systems into balance.

Cold water on your skin stimulates nerve endings below the surface of your skin so they transmit messages to your organs affecting your heart rate, your breathing, even your thinking. Cold water on the skin also communicates with messenger molecules—hormone-like substances including cytokines, substance P, and endorphins—which in turn act on different parts of your body. These tiny messenger molecules connect everything in your body to everything else. Cold water drives the blood to your inside organs by clamping down the blood vessels of the skin; this is why your skin will look pale after a cold-water treatment. But driving the blood inside makes it move faster and supplies inner organs such as the heart, brain, and kidneys with more blood. Better blood supply means swifter, more balanced body functions. Thus, cold water improves regulation, putting the thermostat—and other "stats"—on normal instead of overdrive or slow. In this way, regular cold showers will help you to be less susceptible to cold hands and feet, for instance. Cold showers also make low blood pressure come up and high blood pressure come down. Cold water has been called the *master harmonizer.*

But the effects of cold water do not end here. After you are done with the cold application, the blood returns with a vengeance into the skin, giving you a nice rosy sheen but without loss of heat that happens after a hot bath. Cold water is the *great invigorator* because it renders you immune to the vagaries of the weather by keeping your physiological responses in training.

Warm and Cold Water Work Differently on Your Body

If you plunge one part of your body—say, your arms—into warm water in a sink, your bodily response will be different than if the water were cold. If you slowly raise the temperature of your arm bath by adding hot water from a faucet every so often, the body's warmth response will be even more pronounced. How does warm water act on your body?

The Warmth Response

If you dunk your arms into warm water, you will respond in three stages. First, there will be increased blood flow to your arms. Then, within a short time, more blood will flow not only into your arms but also into your chest. Why? Because your chest—mainly your lungs and your heart—is connected to your arms by a complicated feedback loop of nerve reflexes. In a similar way, if you took a warm footbath, it would affect your head. These distant relationships, still a basic principle of medicine today, were recognized by Sebastian Kneipp. Lastly, if the arm bath lasts long enough and the temperature of the water remains warm, you will experience warmth and increased circulation in your whole body. When you pull your arms out of the water, the circulation of the blood in your arms will slowly return to normal.

Hot water increases metabolism; it makes bodily functions faster. It especially speeds up your heartbeat and deepens your breathing. But, paradoxically, it also has a calming, sedating effect. It lowers blood pressure by pulling blood into the skin vessels. You can see how rosy you look when you are coming out of a hot bath. Hot baths are best taken around bedtime. Because all your blood lingers at the surface, you lose heat faster, and shivering might occur afterward. For that reason, every hot bath should end with a short cold gush or shower to close the pores of your skin.

Water therapy uses the connection between the arms and the chest especially for treating high blood pressure and respiratory diseases like asthma and bronchitis. A warm footbath followed by a short cold gush is used to treat the onset of a head cold.

The Cold Response

If, in contrast, you immerse your arms in cold water, immediately the blood flow to the skin is greatly reduced, and your arms will look pale, as I described earlier. Within a few minutes after you pull your arms out of the cold water, the blood will return to the skin with more vigor than before, and your arms will look rosy and blushed. A feeling of comfortable warmth will fill your arms. This is the phase of *rubor*—the Latin word for reddening of the skin.

If you do this experiment on your own by taking a full bath, you will observe that after warmth exposure, your body will slowly return from hot to normal, whereas after cold exposure, there is a fast warming-up phase and then, slowly, the body will return to normal.

Why these different responses to warmth and cold? Cold is the greater danger, so your body's answer is swift and thorough. Also, when the body is too warm, there is not much choice, short of panting or jumping into cold water. All you can do is open the capillaries in your skin and your extremities to let the warmth dissipate. And that takes time.

The cold response is more like an alarm reaction, so it will activate more regulatory systems in your body. During the years of our evolution from reptiles (or their forerunners) to mammals, the cold response was the new invention. Cold water stimulates your body to create heat by itself—and that is a healthy occurrence.

Five Rules for Safe and Effective Cold-Water Treatments

If you have any doubts about your tolerance for cold water, check with your doctor first. For any cold-water treatments, please follow these five cautionary rules:

1. **Never use ice-cold water for any cold-water treatment.** Sebastian Kneipp's cold water means water of 55°F to 68°F (13°C to 20°C). "Spring cold" is the term he uses for even colder water of 50°F to 59°F (10°C to 15°C), which might give an extra blissful jolt to your soul and your immune system.

    If in the winter the water comes out of the faucet colder, just decrease the exposure time. If you live in a warm area like California or Florida, the way to deal with warmish water is to prolong the exposure time. Another trick is not to towel dry but simply let the water evaporate from your body before you dress.

2. **Never do a cold-water treatment on a cold body or body part.** The cold response—warm, cold, warmer—can happen only in a warm body. If you are cold to begin with, this therapy will not work. If after due time (usually within a few minutes) you still feel cold after a cold-water treatment, your body has shown that it was not able to create its own natural heat. Either it was too cold to start with, or it lacked energy. In any case, you have to take measures so that your body becomes warm again. You can accomplish that by taking a warm footbath, a warm bath, or a warm shower or by getting dressed and then taking a vigorous walk or engaging in other exercise.

3. **Go at your own pace.** Pace yourself, based on your physical condition and the amount of stimuli you can tolerate. As much as you might be excited by reading this book and wanting to try water therapy on the spot, be warned: Young and healthy

people might be able to start by simply taking a short cold shower, especially during the summertime or in one of the warmer states. Less vigorous people might have to start with a slower approach by trying a cold gush to their feet, hands, and face and gradually working their way up to their whole body. Elderly and feeble people should start with a short whole-body wash with a slightly wrung cold facecloth in front of the sink. For very sick people, a cold wash of just one body part—for instance, the back to prevent pneumonia—should be enough of a stimulus.

4. **Every person is different.** The cold stimulus should be as mild as possible so it doesn't weaken your body, but as strong as necessary to induce your own production of natural heat. For every person, the exposure time might be different, because everyone is different.

In a *Kur* (spa) setting, physicians allow for about three to four weeks before patients reach a whole-body cold treatment. Some elderly and weakened people may never reach that goal but do very well with arm and foot baths and cold washings.

People react differently to the same application, depending on season, weather, time of day, and state of mind (nervous, relaxed) and body (tired, hungry, sick). After a cold shower, you should feel warm and invigorated. If you feel cold, rewarm yourself immediately with a warm bath or shower, ending it with a much shorter cold gush than before. You can also warm up yourself with some exercises. A sensation of cold that lasts for hours is a drain on your body instead of an invigorating stimulus.

However distinct the reactions are in one person at different times, the contrasts in different individuals are, of course, even more striking. Research done in the century after Sebastian Kneipp confirms that your constitution is a predictor of how you will react to cold water. The acral rewarming time (how long it takes your fingertips to get warm again after

CATEGORIES OF BODY TYPES USED IN EUROPEAN NATURAL MEDICINE

- **Asthenic** people (slim, small bones, insignificant muscles) tend to have cold fingers, toes, hands, and feet. They benefit from toning with cold applications but need a slow start. Asthenic people often have low blood pressure, and hot baths may lower their blood pressure even more, making them tired and dizzy. Cold showers and moderate exercise will strengthen them.
- **Athletic** people (tall, big bones, significant muscles) have a tendency to sweat. If not "moved" adequately, they will be liable to obesity, but if they exercise, their muscle bulk creates heat. So they need cooling and vigorous movements. They do not need the extra heat of a hot bath.
- **Pycnic** people (medium stature with more fat than muscles) are disposed to obesity with metabolic diseases like diabetes mellitus, high blood pressure, high blood fats, heart attack, and stroke. They respond well to cold-water treatments to get them going but may also benefit from hot baths to increase their metabolism. Exercise will do them good.

your arms have been submerged in cold water for different lengths of time) has been used to measure such constitutional differences.

Of course, people are most often mixtures of body types; they rarely come in a pure form. Find out for yourself what is good for you. The authority over your own body and your own well-being lies in your own hands. Therefore, body type classifications such as the ones in the box can only be a first guiding step. The goal will always be to leave behind these first approaches and find out who you really are and what you really need. You are different at different times of the day, in different seasons, and in different moods. You need to listen to what your body and your mind need *in the present moment*, from hour to hour, day to day, season to season.

Stop any application as soon as you notice that it is not good for you. It might be that a slightly modified water treatment would work better for you. Try to figure out what is best for your body.

5. **Treatments should not be stressful or hurried.** It is better to skip a treatment than to rush. This seems to be a self-evident rule, but I'm including it because all too often we overdo things. Yes, even healthy things can be overdone if they become just another stressor in your life.

Balance is key to good health, and cold-water therapy is a powerful technique for achieving that balance. You can do cold-water therapy in the comfort of your home and create a peaceful haven right in your own bathroom. Move on to Chapter 3 to discover how to enhance the experience of cold-water therapy by transforming your bathroom into a serene, healing spa.

TRANSFORMING YOUR BATHROOM INTO A HEALING WATER SPA

Your bathroom is your private haven, and you can make it into a place of relaxation and renewal. You can turn even a boring utility room into your very own spa by creating a room all your own with posters on the walls, shells or beautiful stones on bookshelves, or whatever artwork you like. Ocean, river, and lake views lend themselves to the tranquility of a spa, but other nature themes work as well. Having plenty of hooks and bookshelves in a bathroom is useful for keeping the room organized and for making sure you have calming, nurturing reading material at your fingertips.

Here are a few suggestions to help create a peaceful, healing atmosphere for your personal spa:

- **Paint your bathroom in your favorite color.** Pastels always work; be careful with vivid colors. Red excites and increases anger—just the opposite of what you want from your bathroom. Blue is cool and soothes but should not be used in a cold, dark room. Yellow is warm and cheerful. Green heals and nourishes. Violet soothes and has a meditative quality as long as it is not too dark. Pink smiles at you. And then there always is white. White works well with plants and wicker and the numerous objects that can center you—for example, plants, shells, rocks, and beads. (My bathroom, by the way, is white.)

- **Invest in a wall- or ceiling-mounted instant heater, activated by a string.** If you shiver in your bathroom, you won't want to spend time there. Do not use space heaters that stand on the floor; the danger of electrocution is too high.
- **Keep your enlightening literature—books and magazines—on a shelf at hand.** Make your new home spa time a time for reflections and insights.
- **Use candles, plants, and occasional incense to help you relax.** Fragrant candles and certain wicks pose a health risk. Better stick to unscented candles and get the fragrance from a drop of essential oil in the bath—whichever one is most relaxing and pleasing for you. Incense, as nice as it smells, also poses some risk to your lungs; use it sparingly. And always be aware of the hazards of open fire.
- **Plants bring life into your bathroom spa and freshen the air.** Ferns, bamboo, and philodendron tolerate dark conditions and thrive in the moist atmosphere of a bathroom. So do *Ficus benjamina* and variegated *Aglaonema*— but they might outgrow the space. Think tropical in the bathroom: palms, colored *Peperomia*, *Spathophyllum*, or African violets.
- **A mirror makes the room look bigger and gives sparkle to the mood in the room.** Not only will a mirror enhance the room's physical attributes, but it will also help you learn to love your body—from the inside and outside. If you don't like your body, work on a more accepting attitude. Look into the mirror every day and learn to embrace yourself and your body. Your body is what you've got to live with. One perspective: we don't have our bodies very long, but our souls soar for eternity.

- **Get terry cloth towels in a color you enjoy.** Mine are all shades of green, one of my favorite colors. You can buy towels at low cost at an outlet store. Mine have minor faults, but they still make me happy. For the water therapy practices in this book, you will need a loofah or natural brush and at least twenty-four facecloths. Try to get the bargain ones in a color you love, but don't scrimp on the number. A facecloth should be used only once before it goes in the laundry.
- **Essential oils, shampoos, lotions, and bath oils are nice but can be expensive.** If you concoct them yourself from the kitchen and the garden, you save money. On a personal note, I have been using the cheapest shampoo plus conditioner for twenty years, and my hair looks healthy. Healthy looking hair and skin come mostly from the inside. So buy an inexpensive shampoo and make sure you rinse it out very thoroughly, because most preserving ingredients are not that healthy to start with, even in expensive shampoos. For lotion, I use olive oil—the very same I use for cooking. Bath oils are special formulations that keep oil and water mixed, as opposed to having the oil just floating on the surface, and are useful for that purpose.

Other Essentials for Your Home Spa

Your bathtub or shower should have handrails and a nonslip mat for safety. Other niceties in the bathroom include a terry cloth robe with slippers and a sturdy place to sit.

The outfitting of the room ultimately is not as important as the activities inside. Sebastian Kneipp made do with the Danube River—and he had to hike there.

The bathroom should be warm at about 62°F to 72°F (17°C to 22°C), and your bed should be warm if you do a cold treatment in the evening. If necessary, warm your bed with a warm water bottle or a microwavable beanbag, but take it out before you lie down. You want to create your own natural heat after the cold stimulus.

BATHROOM BLISS: AN AYURVEDIC OIL BATH

The healing and soothing ayurvedic oil bath comes from the ancient Indian and ayurvedic medical system. The practice, which takes about thirty minutes, rehydrates and re-oils your skin, keeps your skin young and smooth, soothes the winter itch, and takes the bad-hair days out of winter.

You will need about a cup of oil. I use olive oil, although the original ayurvedic recipe calls for sesame oil (the same as you use for kitchen purposes). You can heat the oil in the microwave, using a microwave-proof container. Start at 20 seconds on full power; you always can add time if needed. Or heat the oil on the stove (use a small pot in a bigger pot filled with water). Be extremely careful not to burn yourself. Or you can remove the lid from a small glass bottle of oil, place the bottle in a pot of water, and slowly heat it to the desired temperature—it should feel nice and warm.

Make sure your bathroom is warm and comfortable. Play some soothing music in the background. Stand naked in the dry shower on a towel. Rub the warm oil into your skin lavishly from head to toe. Include your scalp and your hair. Do not worry: it is a feast even for longer hair. Include your face, your ears, your toes, and all the creases, crooks, and crannies of your body.

Let your skin absorb the oil for at least ten minutes. While you wait, do some gentle stretching. But be careful—you now are as slippery as a wet fish.

Take a warm shower, and shampoo your hair twice. Do not use soap on your body because you want your skin to get all the benefit of the oil bath. End with your usual short cold shower. Towel off (the towel needs to go in the laundry afterward). You can also take an oil bath just for your hands; I like it after garden work.

For most skin diseases, this treatment is very soothing. Confer with your physician if you have open sores. Also make sure the oil does not contain ingredients to which you are allergic.

Whether you are in the shower, at the sink, or in the bathtub, your bathroom can be transformed into a healing sanctuary that helps alleviate a variety of health conditions. See Chapter 8 for step-by-step water treatments for specific health problems. Use the elements we discussed above to create a personal and peaceful bathroom—tranquil and inviting. In the next chapter, you'll learn about one particular area in your bathroom—the shower—and the simple techniques that make the ordinary shower a powerful healing tool.

CHAPTER 4

IN THE SHOWER

Begin with a Cold Wash

A cold wash is useful for beginners and for the sick or elderly, and it is a good alternative to the cold shower. It takes about two minutes to do. All you need is a clean washcloth, a source of cold water, and a towel. The washcloth should be changed after each use.

Stand in the shower or bathtub or on a towel in front of the sink. If you are standing in the tub, begin by holding each foot for a few seconds under running water. In front of the sink, if you are flexible, you can hold one foot at a time under the running water. If not, step into a basin with cold water. Wring out a facecloth with cold water, and wash yourself from the face down. Do not use soap.

Towel off your feet and body creases; let the rest of your body air-dry. Alternatively, do not towel off at all after the cold wash; just retire to bed moist, as Sebastian Kneipp recommended.

CAUTION: You should not perform a cold wash if you have:

- Open wounds
- Cold feet (warm them up first in a basin with warm/hot water)
- Acute urogenital diseases
- Acute lower-back pain
- Acute sciatica

Cold Shower

There is no better way to start the day or invigorate your body than a simple cold shower of less than a minute after your customary hot shower. Besides a towel, all you need is a shower or a showerhead in a tub. Sebastian Kneipp, of course, scoffed at the towel: he would just get into his clothes wet and run himself dry. The method described here is a modified version of Sebastian Kneipp's cold-water gushes, adjusted to our times and equipment.

Start with your usual shower. Of course, a warm or hot shower is a wonderful way to relax and get clean. I do not recommend soap; it destroys the slightly acidic pH balance of your skin. In fact, soap is largely unnecessary. How dirty can you be if you take a shower every day (unless you have a really dirty job)? But I know that is not the American way! Also, use a rubber mat to avoid slipping whenever you are in the tub or shower.

After your warm shower, step out of the stream, and turn the handle on cold (as cold as possible—no cheating!). Always begin with your feet. Hold them in the cold flow. Next, do the same with your hands. Then splash your face. That's it for your first time. Easy, wasn't it? The next time you take a shower, start again with your feet and let the water run up to your knees. Then splash your hands and face. In a few days, you will have reached belly button, chest, shoulders, neck, and scalp. But you will always start at the feet. The cold water on your skin sends blood rushing inside your body, where it nourishes your brain, heart, and other internal organs. So initially, your skin will look pale.

Now towel off and get dressed. Within minutes, your pale skin will turn pink, because blood will be flushing back in by a reactive opening of the floodgates of your skin's blood vessels. The cascade of healthy and normal self-regulation will set in and will work in your body long after you have started your day. Your immune system will work better, your mood will get a lift, your breathing will be less shallow, your muscles will feel stronger, and so on. On a molecular level, you will achieve a new balance. As a whole person, you will feel better—and you'll be healthier.

If after a few minutes you are not snugly warm everywhere, especially if your feet or hands stay cold, put them into a warm bath for five to ten minutes, until they feel warm. End with a very short cold exposure (just seconds)—to close the pores, as we say in German. Another way to rewarm your body is with a short rub-down of your skin—excluding the face—with a loofah, a brush, or a rough towel to get your circulation going. Or do some light exercises such as whirling your arms and jumping in place. Next time, shorten your cold shower. If, again, you cannot get warm afterward, you might not be ready for cold showers; try a cold wash first (see the beginning of the chapter).

One cold shower feels great, but its effect is limited. However, if you repeat it day after day, you will see results, the way the steady drops of water carve a canyon. Your skin will glow. You'll feel alive and ready to tackle the stresses in your life, your hair will grow stronger, and you'll get colds and infections less often. Of course, it is much easier to start this program in summer and fall, when the tap water is naturally warmer than in winter and spring. (In February, it is so cold that I scream—but I take my cold shower anyway.) Of course, the cold shower can also be used without the warm part, especially when you are hot after work, from a workout, or just from oppressive heat. But *never take a cold shower on a cold body.*

If you find the cold shower too cold the first few times, try these tips:

- **Don't think cold**—just do it. The less you think about it, the easier it gets.
- **Before turning the handle to cold, turn it to hot** for a few seconds—to very hot. That will make you want to get to the cold part fast.
- **Breathe out** while immersing in the cold water. I have no idea why it works—but it does.

- **Take a very, very short cold shower**—a second for the front, a second for the back—and increase the time slowly. Remember, more isn't necessarily better!
- **Take your time** to work up from your feet to your scalp—every day a little higher. You can give yourself a whole month to achieve the final goal. You are only aiming for twenty to thirty seconds. Listen to your body: if you feel cold when you get out of the shower, you overdid it. If you do it right, you will feel on top of the world.
- **Try different times of the day.** Young and vigorous people might be able to start with a cold shower after their warm morning shower. If you have a hard time in the morning, try the early afternoon. Morning is the time of warming up for the body; and if you do not have enough of your own body heat, you can get used to cold showers better if you take them after noon.

CAUTION: Do not use this treatment if you have:

- Raynaud's (a condition where the hands and/or feet turn white with cold exposure)
- Hardening of the arteries (peripheral vascular disease, angina, cerebral vascular disease)
- Acute urogenital diseases (such as a urinary tract infection, acute prostatitis)
- Acute lower-back pain or sciatica

When in doubt, consult your physician.

People of asthenic (slim) constitution—like myself—should not overdo any cold-water treatment. For instance, during the warm seasons, I take two cold showers, in the morning and evening. But in winter my body tolerates only one, in the morning; in the evening a cold wash (see the beginning of this chapter) has to do. Observe yourself, and find out what you need. Muscular or overweight types might tolerate more and longer cold showers.

Water Temperatures

Water comes in different forms: liquid, gas, solid—water, steam, ice. Hydrotherapy (water therapy) uses all three forms, within a wide range of temperatures. But most of the time, we use the water just as it comes out of the tap. Tap water is not necessarily the healthiest form of water. Take every opportunity to get water at its purest: walk barefoot at the beach or in a creek, stand under a waterfall, or swim in a pristine lake; they are the real thing and will teach you to appreciate this life-sustaining element. But for every day, water from your tap is an underrated boon.

Here is a list of the approximate water temperatures referred to in this book:

Very cold	32°F–56°F	0°C–13°C	Icy water
Cold	56°F–65°F	13°C–18°C	Spring water
Cool	65°F–75°F	18°C–24°C	Tap water
Neutral	75°F–94°F	24°C–34°C	Tepid (lukewarm) water
Warm	95°F–104°F	35°C–40°C	Body-temperature water
Hot	Above 104°F	Above 40°C	Hot water

Alternating Hot and Cold Shower

When you take an alternating hot and cold shower, always start warm and end cold. You may go through as many cycles as you wish, but the more you do, the more exhausting it will be. So this is best done in the evening. But if you have to function after a night without sleep, this is a rather drastic measure to get you going again. In this case, only do two cycles.

This practice treats muscle pain, acts as a shock to the system, reviving body and spirit, and helps you get used to cold showers. The warm shower eliminates toxins; the cool shower acts against inflammation.

CHAPTER 5

IN THE BATHTUB

The bathtub can be an incredible place for healing and reju-
venation. While alternating between cold and hot showers
is much easier, especially in this fast-paced world, you will be
amazed at the health benefits of taking a long, relaxing bath. But
a bath may be more than just any old bath—different types of
baths can address a variety of health conditions:

Health Conditions	Healing Treatments
Fatigue	Warm bath
Stress	Warm bath
Lack of energy	Cold sitz bath (happy half bath)
Tired feet	Warm footbath
Tired legs	Cold knee/leg gush, cold sitz bath
Muscle and joint pain	Warm saltwater bath or mud bath
Dry, itchy skin	Warm saltwater bath or mud bath
Varicose veins	Cold knee/leg gush, cold sitz bath
Circulation problems	Warm saltwater bath or mud bath

| Fever | Fever-reducing bath |
| Many conditions | Warm-to-hot herbal bath |

Warm Bath—Preferably with Herbs

A warm bath is the epitome of pampering, a reminder of child-hood when we were loved and coddled and put to bed after a warm bath. Now grown up, you can treat yourself royally with a warm bath. You can also add herbs, essential oils, or specialized bath formulas to the water. Use a warm bath whenever you feel tired, achy, disappointed, stressed, negative, or exhausted.

Make sure your bathroom is comfortably warm before getting in the tub. Your water temperature should be 97°F to 104°F (36°C to 40°C). Higher temperatures are more strenuous for the heart; you begin sweating on your forehead. The best temperature for you is a matter of preference and contraindications. Herbal sub-stances work better with higher temperatures, but do not boil yourself. The total bath time, including rubbing moisturizing oils or creams on your skin afterward, takes about thirty minutes to an hour.

A warm bath has many healing properties. It increases well-being and vitality and promotes recuperation after an illness, stimulating receptors on and/or in the skin, communicating with your nervous system. It also dilates your blood vessels—first in your skin, then also deeper in your body—and increases the activ-ity of your gastrointestinal tract, relaxing tight muscles, reliev-ing soreness, and producing endorphins in our brain—our very own substances to give us a "high" and relieve pain. A bath also reduces pain by activating receptors in the spinal cord (the reason why underwater birth is less painful). And a bath can mend bones and reduce fever (see the section on fever-reducing baths later in this chapter).

For the skin, a warm bath stimulates circulation and heals. It also decreases the blood pressure transiently (although it does *not* have the balancing effect on high blood pressure of regular cold showers), which makes you sleepy and ready for bed. So have your bed warmed up before you take a bath.

Using Bath Herbs

For many health conditions, specific herbs can be used as essential oils or as a tea (also called an infusion) to heal. For essential oils, you usually use three to six drops or follow the instructions on the bottle. As a tea or infusion added to the bathwater, you need enough of the herbs for several cups of tea. Make the tea according to the instructions in Chapter 18 and pour it in the tub. An alternative is to fill a clean cotton sock with herbs and let the hot water from the tap run over it and into the bathtub.

WARM HERBAL BATHS FOR SKIN DISEASE

A bath you take for your skin should not be warmer than 97°F (36°C), since the protective action of the bathing ingredients might be undermined by too-high water temperature. These baths are an exception to the emulsifier combination. The idea here is that the oil swims on the surface generously and is clinging to your skin while you move in and out of the bath through the surface, giving your skin a much thicker coat than from bath oil. For herbs to use, refer to the specific skin problems listed.

Herbs for Specific Conditions

If you have one of the following conditions, use any of the suggested herbs for the condition in a warm bath:

- **Aches and pains, muscle spasms, sciatica, arthritis, bursitis:** chamomile, comfrey, eucalyptus, hayflowers (grass, weeds, and flowers from a meadow, mown and dried), jasmine, juniper, lavender, menthol, orange essential oil, pine, rose, sweet almond oil, wintergreen
- **Aging:** apple cider vinegar, jasmine, rose
- **Anxiety, anger, worries:** chamomile, jasmine, rose. Rose petals, fresh from the garden, are a wonderful additive to your bath.
- **Bone pain, broken bones:** comfrey
- **Circulation:** comfrey
- **Colds and flu, bronchitis, congestion:** camphor, eucalyptus, evergreens, menthol, tea tree oil, thyme
- **Constipation:** Any warm bath (with or without herbs) will help constipation because the water pressure alone of a full bath presses on your abdomen and massages your bowels. Also, because warm water stimulates the parasympathetic nerve paths, it hastens passage through the system. But do not take a bath with a full stomach.
- **Eczema:** evening primrose, kelp, olive oil, soybean oil (For more on preparing warm baths for skin conditions, see the sidebar.)
- **Fatigue, exhaustion:** apple cider vinegar, jasmine, rose, sage, spirulina, wintergreen
- **Female pains:** clary, jasmine, marjoram, rose
- **Hair troubles:** sage
- **Impending cold:** lavender, tea tree oil
- **Mild varicose veins:** arnica, calendula (Severe varicose veins need cold water; hot baths are contraindicated.)
- **Skin inflammation:** chamomile, horsetail, kelp, yarrow

- **Skin that is dry:** bath oil, olive oil, yogurt (plain natural, a small cup)
- **Skin that itches:** menthol, thyme
- **Skin that itches and has open sores:** bran, kelp, oak bark extract, oats
- **Sleeplessness:** hops, lemon balm, lemon grass, valerian
- **Stress:** chamomile, jasmine, lavender, rose
- **Toxicity:** apple cider vinegar

Happy Half Bath (Cold Sitz Bath)

A happy half bath (also called cold sitz bath) stimulates and energizes, reduces inflammation, and is a great way to start the day. It is also refreshing in the middle of a hot, humid summer day or when one cannot sleep during an oppressive night. Other benefits include helping with depression, fighting fatigue, and lowering fever (for adults only). It also shrinks and soothes hemorrhoids, boosts fertility in men and women, softens irritability, and counteracts flabbiness of the lower part of your body. It is a great tool to overcome procrastination and lack of motivation. This was one of Sebastian Kneipp's favorite invigorating treatments.

Moreover, a cold sitz bath reduces frequent infections, improves skin problems, especially acne and a sallow skin color, is excellent for treating varicose veins, improves circulation, and helps relieve general asthenia or weakness (use with caution in the elderly and sick!). It is excellent for treating chronic prostatitis (avoid in acute prostatitis and urinary tract infections) and often brings relief from rheumatism and inflamed joints. It also helps combat sleeplessness. Instead of tossing and turning, take a happy half bath in the middle of the night, and return to bed (but make sure you don't get cold feet).

Fill your bathtub with cold water from the faucet, at a temperature of about 64°F to 68°F (18°C to 20°C). The water may reach your navel, but this treatment also works well with just two inches of water—enough to cover your private parts. Adjust to the happy half bath slowly by having only a few inches of cold water in the tub for the first time. Sit down for a few seconds, not longer than twenty to thirty seconds. Towel off, dress, and then move. Hardy people can try this as a full cold bath, too—but only for a few seconds.

Wonder why the same treatment is good for waking you up (in the morning) and putting you to sleep (in the evening)? Cold water enhances the natural mode of your body according to the circadian rhythm: in the morning, wakefulness, and in the evening, sleepiness.

For whatever reason you take the happy half bath, it leaves you with a feeling of exhilaration and renewed vitality. In the long run (after about six weeks), it rejuvenates you and strengthens your immune system.

CAUTION: Do not use this treatment if you have:

- An acute cold
- Acute back pain
- An acute urinary tract infection

Cold Massage Bath

The cold massage bath is a variation on the happy half bath. You use the same water temperature and depth, but in addition, you vigorously and rapidly scrub yourself with a loofah or a brush, or knead your whole body while you are in the water. The massage stimulates the circulation. This bath is very good if done on sick and feeble persons. Avoid long exposures though.

Warm Footbath

What could be more relaxing than taking a footbath after a long day on your feet—standing at work, treading asphalt while shopping, or after an arduous hike? A footbath is easy to prepare, less effort than a whole bath, and still revitalizes not only your feet, but distant parts of your body as well. You can sit on the edge of your bathtub and dangle your feet in the warm water, or you can use a foot basin. Don't forget to end with a very short cold gush to your feet.

You might want to combine a footbath not only with a pedicure but also with a gentle foot massage. Because every part of your body corresponds to a part of your foot, your whole body benefits from a foot massage.

This bath wakes up tired feet, warms cold feet, increases circulation throughout your body, calms your nerves, and soothes headaches. Because of a direct "line" between feet and head, it relieves congestion and may even stop a cold if you take the footbath right at the onset. The warm water keeps feet beautiful and softens corns and calluses. Taken before bedtime, a warm footbath promotes sleepiness because the worst sleep robbers are cold feet.

There are no cautions or contraindications for a warm footbath.

Cold Knee/Leg Gush

The cold knee/leg gush is an easy practice that instantly revives tired, heavy legs and helps with varicose veins. Starting at your feet and moving up slowly, let cold water from the tub faucet or from a removable showerhead run over your knees and legs for about one minute. If you don't want to do this in a bathtub, go outside and use your garden hose! But beware of high water pressure—a gentle flow is what you want.

CAUTION: Do not use this treatment if you have:

- Cold feet
- Acute urogenital diseases
- Acute lower-back pain
- Narrowing (atherosclerosis) of leg arteries
- Raynaud's

Warm Saltwater Bath

Saltwater baths are also called ocean therapy (thalassotherapy). It would be nice to swim at the beach, but you can also indulge yourself at home. Bathing in saltwater works like a diuretic, detoxifies your body, increases blood flow to the skin and circulation in general, relieves muscle and joint pains, and soothes and sedates dry and itchy skin. In fact, it heals or improves many chronic skin conditions.

For a salt bath, empty about half a cup of any of these types of salt into a warm bath: table salt, Dead Sea salt (available in health food stores and vitamin shops), Epsom salts (with magnesium sulfate), or seaweed powder. Some of the beneficial minerals will be absorbed through the skin. Spend about thirty minutes soaking in the tub.

Salt baths are more strenuous than simple or herbal baths. Therefore, plan on going to bed afterward. And do not use them often—not more than once a week.

CAUTION: Do not use this treatment if you have:

- High blood pressure
- Heart disease
- Kidney problems

If you have open skin sores, the salt will sting but might also promote healing.

Warm Mud Bath

The warm mud bath is an ancient practice that has benefits similar to saltwater baths. Its results very much depend on the ingredients of the mud you use. Always read the label before you purchase your mud, which you can find in many health food stores. You might want to try Dead Sea mud first, because it is famous for its powerful healing properties. Follow the directions on the package. In addition to the mud you choose for your bath, you will need a facecloth, a towel, and some good lotion or oil for after the bath. I prefer plain olive oil sprinkled with a few drops of an essential oil like myrrh, rose, oregano, or thyme.

Sitting in mud is a weird experience, right up there with bathing in champagne or donkey's milk (neither of which I have tried—yet). The slightly higher viscosity immediately slows down your movements and instills a languid mood. Most people enjoy getting dirty playfully. Keep your head out of the mud—but you can use a facecloth to apply mud to your face (sparing the area around the eyes). When you are done, drain the mud-water. Rinse off with warm water (a handheld showerhead is ideal for this, but you can also use running water from the tub faucet or transfer to the shower stall). As always, end with a short cold shower.

Another way to apply mud is as a thick paste (stir in some warm water until it has the consistency of cake dough) to your whole body, again, sparing the eyes. You do this in the shower and then wait until the paste starts drying or you start itching. This is how the famous mud baths at the Dead Sea are applied. When you are done, rinse yourself carefully with warm water; end with a short cold shower. If you have the time, combine this with a warm oil bath afterward. You will emerge from this spa experience glowing with health and beauty.

As you can imagine, a good mud bath will make a mess in your tub. Clean up right after the mud bath, before it cakes.

CAUTION: Do not use this treatment if you have:

- High blood pressure
- Heart disease
- Kidney problems
- Open skin sores

Fever-Reducing Bath

A fever-reducing bath lowers the body temperature in a mild and nonchemical way. It is for people with fever—especially small children—who are at the height of their fever, feel very warm, have warm hands and feet, and look rosy or even red.

The temperature of this bath should be about 2°F below the body temperature. Immerse yourself or your child into the water. Slowly add colder water. Conclude the bath immediately at any sign of worsening or stress. Finish the bath in twenty minutes or whenever the bather feels cold. Never leave a sick person in a bath without supervision—not even for a second!

Towel off, and quickly return to bed. Cover yourself or your child well. There will be a lot of sweating, which is the desired effect. The fever should be lowered by about 2°F. This kind of bath in this situation is to be done only once a day, preferably in the afternoon to get the benefit of the circadian rhythm, since the afternoon is the cooling-down period.

CAUTION: Do not use this treatment if you have:

- A fever that is still rising
- Cold hands and/or feet
- Pale skin

These are all signs of centralization, which is a sign that the body already is in severe stress.

The Warm-to-Hot Bath

You might add hotter water to the bath while you are in the tub; that is called a warm-to-hot bath. It has an even stronger effect. Thirty minutes generally is enough luxuriating in a tub. Always end your warm-to-hot bath with a short cold gush to your whole body or a short cold shower to close the pores.

The warm-to-hot bath, as you can comfortably tolerate it, stimulates metabolism, making it ideal for obesity, diabetes, gout, and all diseases that stem from toxic overload. It is also deodorizing and antiseptic. The pressure of the water induces the blood to return to the heart, which stimulates the heart and increases the heartbeat. Therefore, if you have a weak heart, you should never have the water level higher than your navel.

If you use herbs or essential oils, the aromatherapy affects your nervous system via your sense of smell. Inhaling the essential oils works on your whole respiratory system, from the sinuses to deep in your lungs. Some of the oil components are taken up through your skin, having an overall effect on your body.

CAUTION: Do not use this treatment if you have:

- Fever: a warm herbal bath might help you in the beginning of a cold or flu, but not any more when your body's immune defense already has created a higher temperature to fight the germs. Then, any addition of warmth might lead to overburdening of your heart.
- Congestive heart failure and uncontrolled high blood pressure: however, it's possible you could tolerate a not-too-warm bath not exceeding the level of your navel (so-called half bath); discuss this with your physician.
- Varicose veins, especially if severe.
- Pregnancy: pregnant women should not bathe warmer than their body temperature (98°F), with the water level preferably below the navel.
- Recurrent urinary tract infections after a full bath: besides being very meticulous in cleaning your bathtub, there is not much one can do except for taking showers instead of baths.

Healthy elderly patients should limit the water level of their bath to not more than a three-quarter bath, that is, water up to the lower part of the breastbone.

CHAPTER 6

AT THE SINK

Not as impressive as your shower and bathtub, the sink, nevertheless, can bring wonderful relief from a variety of ailments. Simple procedures done right at your kitchen or bathroom sink can relieve any of the following conditions:

Health Conditions	Healing Treatments
Bad gums or teeth	Cold mouth rinse
High blood pressure	Cold arm bath
Stuffy nose	Saltwater nose rinse
Tension headaches	Cold head dunk
Lung afflictions	Cold arm bath
Indecisiveness	Cold head dunk
Carpal tunnel syndrome	Cold arm bath
Tired eyes, poor vision, wrinkles	Cold eye wash

Cold Mouth Rinse

The cold mouth rinse is a practice that comes down to us from Hildegard von Bingen (1098–1179), a medieval nun, herbalist, composer, and stateswoman. Rinsing your mouth with cold water is a good way to invigorate your gums—paramount for healthy teeth. After brushing your teeth or just after eating, rinse your mouth with cold water—the colder, the better. Let the cold water swirl around your teeth. Swish the cold water around in your mouth until it warms up. The first few times, it might feel as if the cold will shatter your teeth. But you will get used to it.

This technique uses no props and has no contraindications or cautions. Enjoy!

Cold Arm Bath

Dunking your arms in cold water reduces high blood pressure, relieves carpal tunnel and repetitive stress syndromes, beautifies hands and nails, and fights the tendency to have cold fingers. It also improves circulation throughout the body but especially in the chest, and therefore improves breathing for people with asthma and chronic bronchitis.

Fill the sink with cold water. Dip both arms into the water above the elbows for up to five minutes.

CAUTION: Do not use this treatment if you have Raynaud's.

Saltwater Nose Rinse

Many years ago, an ENT (ear, nose, and throat) physician suggested sinus surgery for a chronic condition I had had for years. I refused the surgery. Because I was a colleague, he shared an old secret with me, admonishing me never to tell it to patients (and admitted he was afraid to lose patients if word got out about this simple healing measure). But ever since, I have been distributing the "secret" saltwater nose rinse among friends and patients. Only later did I learn that it is an ancient ayurvedic procedure from India.

This is the single best thing I know against a stuffy nose from viruses, allergies, or bacterial infection. Even though this practice is revolting in the beginning, it is worth learning and doing. It cleans the nose of discharge, relieves clogged nasal passages, helps open the eustachian tubes during earaches, reduces allergen and pollen load in hay fever, removes bacteria and viruses, thereby protecting you from colds and epidemics, and shortens the course of the illness. You should do this at least once a day when you don't have a cold; do it more often if your nose is stuffed. During a severe cold, I did it one night about thirty times. Next morning, I had not slept much—but my nose was free, and I was on the way to recovery.

Take a glass of lukewarm water, about cup-size (later, when you will be hardier, it can be cold), and add a quarter of a teaspoonful of kitchen salt or sea salt. Stir and pour some of this saltwater in the hollow of your palm. Lower your head, and suck the water up your nostrils. It will travel down into your mouth. *Do not swallow.* Spit it out. Repeat until all the water has been used.

This procedure sounds awful, and in the beginning, it is just that. But you will not drown, even if it feels like it. Just keep trying. It took me about half a year to do this procedure without sputtering and choking, but it works wonders.

Ayurvedic medicine has developed a little device, a neti pot, to pour the saltwater in your nostrils. But it may break in the sink and is just another thing to clean. I find all you need are your hands and some saltwater.

If you have high blood pressure, avoid taking in extra salt. Rinse your mouth (not your nose) afterward with clear water. Do not swallow the salty phlegm; spit it out.

Be careful not to use too much salt. It will make the inside of your nose burn. Too little salt, by contrast, makes your nose sting. Learning to distinguish the two takes experience. It's better to err on the side of too little salt.

Head Dunk

The head dunk is perfect for treating a tension headache and too much thinking (or computer games). Because it makes a mess of one's hair, this seems to be a guy thing. But its effects are indeed gender-neutral. Students, CEOs, and people who have to make quick decisions might benefit the most from a cold head dunk.

Match the water temperature to the condition you're treating: cold gives your system a refreshing jolt, warm soothes a congested head. A cold head dunk treats headaches (except sinus headache), fatigue, exhaustion, angry or depressive mood, and difficulty making a quick decision. A warm head dunk treats sinus head-aches, head congestion, and a cold—make sure to towel your hair well afterwards, and stay out of drafts. Alternating dunks (always start warm and end cold) help with memory problems, tired face, and hair loss.

Close your eyes, mouth, and nose, and immerse your head in a basin, sink, or bucket filled with water of the desired temperature. On the go, you might just put your head under a faucet and let the cold water run over your head. It works like a mini cold shower. Remain under the water for less than a minute.

CAUTION: Do not use this treatment if you have:

- Eye disease
- Perforated eardrum
- Uncontrolled high blood pressure

Cold Eye Wash

The cold eye wash offers instant relief for tired eyes, helps maintain good vision and good looks longer into old age, tones the skin around the eyes, and reduces irritation, swelling, and inflammation. It also may remove foreign objects.

Bend over the sink. Try to keep your eyes open, and gently pour water in each eye with your hands for a few seconds. Lightly pat down around the eyes to dry; don't rub. If your tap water is too chlorinated or contaminated, use bottled water from a clean cup with a spout. If you want to add herbs like eyebright, you can buy an eyecup in a drugstore.

CAUTION: Make sure you let any herbal infusion cool before you use it in your eyes. Note that most herbs are not suited for use in your eyes. Do not splash hard; be gentle. Do not rub. Be careful with a dubious water supply or if your municipal water is overtreated with chlorine; with any suspicious water resource, use bottled water. The truth is that you can't be 100 percent sure about water. But, definitely, if the water is not meant for consumption, it also should not go into your eyes. Do not use this treatment if you have:

- Any serious eye problems
- Cataracts
- Glaucoma
- Immune deficiency
- Infections

CHAPTER 7

OUTSIDE THE HOME

Your bathroom is your haven for relaxation, but the real water happens outside: the ocean, a brook, a waterfall, a dewy meadow—just help yourself to what nature provides, cleaner and cheaper than the faucet at home. Public facilities afford other water opportunities: pools, saunas, whirlpools, and steam baths. You might even dream of building one in your home. But the most important thing is: never let a water occasion go by unused!

If you want to relieve any of the following conditions outside the home, try the ideas suggested in this chapter:

Health Conditions	Healing Treatments
Stroke, multiple sclerosis (MS), arthritis	Water exercise
Sports injuries, arthritis, stress	Whirlpool
Acne, stress, detoxification, immune training	Sauna
Skin, circulation, and breathing problems	Steam bath
Constipation, immune problems, headaches	Cold-water treading
Tired legs	Cold-water treading
Varicose veins	Cold-water treading

Water Exercise (Pool Gymnastics)

Underwater exercise or movement in a pool can be used when exercising on dry land is painful or difficult, as after a stroke or with arthritis or disabling diseases such as MS. The water should never be cold but pleasurable.

Exercising in the water relieves joints, muscles, and tendons from strain because of relative weightlessness in the water. But the resistance of water is more than ten times that of the air, so you get a good workout for muscles, heart, and lungs. And it is sheer fun!

Water makes exercise possible for people with joint, muscle, bone, and nerve diseases, increasing the range of motion beyond what could be achieved on land. Exercises you can do in the pool or that are offered in classes include aerobics, ball games, jumping, kickboxing, resistance training, swimming, water tai chi, water walking, and Watsu (water shiatsu).

Wear water shoes to prevent slipping, and beware of infections and overexposure to chlorine. Take a thorough shower after each class, always ending cold.

CAUTION: Do not use this treatment if you have:

- Open wounds
- Acute disease
- Fever
- Any contagious infection

Whirlpool or Hot Tub

Whirling water energizes, but it may also drain energy from you because the water in a whirlpool usually is rather hot. Whirlpools and hot tubs are thought of as being relaxing. But of all the water works presented here, they are also the most demanding on the heart. They increase blood return to the heart, which can be invigorating or overwhelming, depending on your heart health. Check with your doctor before using whirling hot water.

Take enough time to enjoy the effects. Rushing through fun does not improve your quality of life. But don't linger more than twenty minutes, especially if the water temperature is much higher than that of your body.

The action of the jet stream relaxes muscles, similar to a massage, and increases your circulation and range of motion in arthritic joints or after trauma and sports injuries. It counteracts cellulite by working fatty tissue—but still is not a substitute for regular exercise and a reasonable dairy-free diet. It also softens scar tissue (apply vitamin E to the skin afterward), detoxifies the body, and cleanses the skin.

Always end with a short cold shower.

CAUTION: Do not use this treatment if you have:

- Heart disease (confer with your physician)
- Open wounds
- Acute disease
- Any contagious infection

Please note that this treatment is not appropriate for pregnant women.

Sauna

In Finland (and the rest of Europe), when families and friends gather for a sauna, everybody is in the nude, children and older folks included. The effect of heat on your body dressed in a bathing suit is different from that in your birthday suit. In the United States, nakedness might pose a problem. Do not push the issue if you or other people do not feel comfortable with nakedness. But give it a try if it is appropriate.

Sauna combines the advantages of sweating and cold-water exposure. It stimulates sweating, cleanses your skin, and opens pores. This is especially helpful as an adjunct treatment for acne. It also detoxifies your body, increases blood circulation, relaxes muscles and mind, relieves stress in a profound way, and eases aches and pains. If you use a sauna regularly, it can prevent colds and improve skin health, mood, and bone density. Saunas are antidepressive and energizing, keeping blood vessels responsive and elastic. They open the respiratory system and may even help in weight loss, but what you lose is mostly water.

In spite of the high sauna temperatures—between 140°F (60°C) downstairs to 208°F (98°C) upstairs—the body can deal with the heat because of the low humidity of the air. Through sweating and the evaporation of the sweat, the body maintains a relatively normal temperature. I usually find that American saunas are kept not as hot as I am used to. Since the heat is higher on the higher benches (the inverse is true for humidity), you should be able to find a position where you feel comfortable with the temperature.

Prepare by taking a warm shower. If your feet are still cold, add a warm footbath before you enter the sauna. Your feet have to be warm.

In the sauna, sit or lie on a towel; dripping sweat makes sitting on the bare wood unhygienic. The optimal time to spend in the hot sauna room is about five to fifteen minutes; maximum is twenty minutes. Leave the sauna immediately if you feel faint or uncomfortable; do not try to tough it out. Skin temperature rises fast and dramatically (to about 104°F), but your core temperature should not rise if you do not overexpose yourself. The invigorating action of the sauna stems from the change in temperatures, not from overheating your body seriously.

After leaving the hot sauna room, walk for a few minutes, preferably outside. This releases more sweat. Before you start to feel cold, have a cold gush, starting with the legs, or enter a cold-water basin up to your chin. Never submerge your head in the cold-water basin. Don't stay more than a minute in the cold—a few seconds will do. Afterward, wrap yourself in a big bath towel or a terry cloth gown, and rest at least twenty to thirty minutes on a recliner before you return to the hot sauna room for the next round.

Do not do more than three sauna rounds. Always rest in between.

Sauna Timetable

5 minutes	Warm shower with short cold shower for cleansing
5 to 15 minutes	First sauna round
5 minutes	Walking (preferably outside in nature)
Less than 1 minute	Cold basin or cold shower (or swim in lake or ocean)
15 to 30 minutes	Resting on a recliner in your bathrobe
5 to 15 minutes	Second sauna round
5 minutes	Walking
Less than 1 minute	Cold basin or cold shower
15 to 30 minutes	Resting
5 to 15 minutes	Third sauna round

5 minutes	Walking
5 to 10 minutes	Final shower to wash hair and groom
Less than 1 minute	Cold basin or cold shower
15 to 30 minutes	Resting

You can see that one can easily spend a whole day in the sauna, especially when you combine it with swimming and exercises. (Never exercise in the hot sauna room; that would strain the heart.) You do not have to do three sauna rounds every time, but never rush through the sauna—that would counteract its entire purpose.

Before you start using the sauna, please confer with your physician to make sure it is safe for you. Also, never enter the sauna with a full stomach or after alcoholic beverages. It is important, however, that you drink plenty of diluted natural juices to replenish your electrolytes.

CAUTION: Do not use this treatment if you have:

- Uncontrolled hypertension
- Heart failure
- Cold feet (with cold feet, always start with a warm footbath)
- Acute urogenital diseases
- Acute lower-back pain

Steam Bath

There are Roman and Russian and Turkish steam baths, as well as other kinds. If you are offered the opportunity to take a steam bath, don't pass it by. Temperatures are around 122°F to 140°F (50°C to 60°C) with very high humidity. Consequently, the steam bath feels very hot. You stay in the steam for about five to ten minutes and then take a break with a short cold shower. Repeat once or twice. The whole process takes an hour; don't rush through it. You can combine it with a sauna: take one or two steam baths and one or two saunas for a total of three to four courses altogether.

A steam bath relaxes and renews, stimulates sweating, increases circulation, cleanses your skin, unclogs your pores, detoxifies your body, increases blood circulation, relaxes muscles, opens stuffed nasal passages, relieves aches and pains, beautifies hair and skin, and helps with asthma and other lung diseases.

CAUTION: Do not engage in a steam bath if you are pregnant.

Cold-Water Treading

In Europe, one finds water-treading basins in spas and public places, and even in private homes and gardens. The best version of this exercise, of course, is to walk barefoot at the beach, in a creek, in a dewy meadow, or on wet pebbles. Cold-water treading is the home version. It refreshes and invigorates. With regular use, it strengthens the immune system, improves and prevents constipation, slows the development of varicose veins, relieves headaches, boosts your mood, and fights fatigue.

Fill a small tub, bowl, basin, or bucket with cold water to a level below your knees. The bottom of the container has to be wide enough so that you can stand in it comfortably. Step into the container, and walk in place. With each step, pull your foot entirely out of the water. Start with a few seconds the first time, or until a very slight pain starts in your feet and legs. Try a few more seconds the next day. Gradually work your way up to several minutes. Have a towel ready on the floor. Step on it. Shake away or brush off most of the moisture, but do not towel off. Walk barefoot or do foot exercises until your feet are dry and warm again.

CAUTION: Do not use this treatment if you have:

- Narrowing of the leg arteries
- Raynaud's
- Open wounds on the feet
- Cold feet
- Urogenital disease
- Acute lower-back pain

CHAPTER 8

WATER TREATMENTS FOR SELECTED HEALTH ISSUES

Water treatments come in many forms—some of them surprising. They are effective in treating any number of health conditions. In addition to those in Chapters 5 through 7, which apply to many situations, the following treatments target particular conditions:

Health Conditions	Healing Treatments
Skin problems	Face masks, facial steam
Sinus problems	Steam inhalation, vaporizer
Stress	Indoor fountain
Insomnia	Wet socks
Impaired circulation, asthma, cellulite	Brushing of the skin
Sore feet, constipation, varicose veins	Walking barefoot
Muscle and joint pain	Compresses

Fever	Cold whole-body wrappings
Respiratory diseases, insomnia	Chest wrappings
Constipation	Warm-water enema

Skin Care with Water

The two main reasons why we wash are to get clean and to moisturize the skin. How to do this right? Remember that beauty comes from the inside. First, drink enough water to keep your skin moisturized from the inside. And eat wholesome foods. Think of fruit and vegetables as carriers of purified water.

When you wash, use plenty of water. Cold is better for your face; hot water can burst tiny vessels in your facial skin leading to unsightly redness (see Chapter 2). Use as little soap as possible. Detergents with a low pH are better than alkaline soap, which destroys the natural acidity of the skin (which lies at a pH of 5.5). Read the labels to determine which soaps have a low pH.

An even gentler abrasive is rolled oats: Make a paste from rolled oats with a few drops of water; rub your face (but not around the eyes). Avoid pulling or picking at your skin. Flush generously with water—first with warm (never hot!), then with cold water.

You don't need a lot of commercial products. Rose water is an old-fashioned tonic for your skin. Witch hazel is an astringent if you have large pores. Don't get it in your eyes. Use creams, oils, and makeup as little as possible. As you get older, you might need some cream, but only use it on areas that seem dry. Do not use it indiscriminately over your whole face. Try Chinese Pearl Cream around the eyes and against wrinkles—you'll find it in Chinese supermarkets and pharmacies. I find it very effective and inexpensive. Expensive body care products do not necessarily guarantee a better outcome.

Face masks and facial steam are especially good for your skin.

Face Masks

Masks improve your complexion within minutes—for instance, if you want to look beautiful for an evening out. Masks nourish, beautify, and moisturize the skin. Rinse them off when your skin feels tight or starts tingling—after ten to twenty minutes. Rinse off the mask immediately if you experience itching, burning, or swelling. Always avoid the eye region where the skin is very delicate.

In general, when applying a face mask, cover your face with the paste, and leave it on until dry. Wash it off with plenty of lukewarm water. Splash with cold water for a final rinse.

Types of Natural Face Masks You Might Want to Try

- Mash cucumber, avocado, and/or aloe (the soft gel from the inside of the leaf).
- Whisk one egg yolk with two teaspoons of honey. Honey closes pores and tightens tired skin. Yolks (or oils) soothe dry skin. Yolks also soothe blotchy skin. Another skin "tightener" is egg white, good for oily skin.
- Make a paste with rolled oats and water—as described previously. Add yogurt for dry skin, water for oily skin, lemon juice for blemishes.
- Stir shredded coconut (preferably fresh) with warm water into a paste. You can also use commercial coconut milk from a can, combining it with avocado, for example, for dry skin.
- Revitalizing masks can be made from cucumbers, strawberries, or grapes.
- Grate carrots; mix with yogurt. Let the mixture stand for half an hour before applying the juice only. This mask is good for treating oily skin but might give your skin a yellowish tinge, which will look like a light tan in brunette people. Blondes should avoid it since it looks unnatural. It washes off after a few days. Plain yogurt, because of its fat contents, is good for treating dry skin.

Facial Steam

Besides making you beautiful, steaming your face is good for your whole respiratory system and is excellent for treating blackheads and acne. It revitalizes a tired face—just the right thing to do before going out in the evening.

Fill a pot or bowl with boiling water and, if you wish, a drop or two of the essential oil of your choice. Drape a towel over your head and the pot, close your eyes, and expose your face to the steam for about ten minutes. Back off if it feels too hot. Inhale slowly through your nose. Afterward, splash your face with cold water to close the pores. If you want to squeeze some blackheads, this is the perfect time since they are softened now. Never squeeze pimples! Apply tea tree oil immediately afterward to prevent infection.

Steam Inhalation/Vaporizer

Inhaling steam, either alone or with herbs, clears out the nose and sinuses in acute and chronic situations. The relief for your breathing will last about five hours. You can use a pot, inhaler, or steam bath (see Chapter 7). Please note that this treatment is not advised for children under ten.

This is done in the same way as the facial steam. Only this time, the focus is on inhaling through the nose (if possible). But this time, add an herb or herbal preparation of your choice, choosing one from the following list. Under the towel, inhale as long as you feel you are getting steam into your lungs. If you can, breathe in through your nose. Breathe in the steam for about fifteen minutes, being careful not to scald yourself.

Use the plain steam, or further the action with any of the following herbs:

- Chamomile (two tea bags)
- Eucalyptus (two drops)

- Lemon essential oil (two drops)
- Linden flower essential oil (two drops)
- Peppermint (two drops essential oil or two tea bags)
- Tea tree oil (two drops)
- Commercial vapor rub (a pea-sized piece)

CAUTION: Do not use this treatment if you have:

- A tendency toward redness in your face from telangiectasias or rosacea
- Allergies to herbal ingredients

Indoor Fountains and Feng Shui

Water is important for more than drinking and bathing. It also is a powerful metaphor for purity, health, transformation, wisdom, and fertility. Dew and clear spring water stand for clarity and secret wisdom. The ebb and flow of the tides symbolize the ups and downs of our lives. To add tranquility and spirituality to your home, bring flowing water indoors with a bubbling fountain and plants, a Chinese misting spring, or a fish tank (goldfish are low maintenance). Or use them all, as I do in my house.

Feng shui, the Chinese art of arranging and harmonizing your home, sees water as the great communicator; there would be no exchange of nutrients between plants and animals and our bodies without the communicating, transporting water. In feng shui philosophy, placing driftwood, shells, pebbles, frog statues, blue marbles, mirrors, and other symbols of water in your house helps to soothe the terrifying water spirits—as in thunderstorm, flooding, monsoon, typhoon, hurricane, tsunami. Whether you believe in the spirits or not, your home will become more beautiful and serene. In addition to serenity, fountains and other sources of water keep air humidity up, which is important for people, pets, plants, and musical instruments. For the Chinese, flowing water also is a symbol of freely flowing material wealth.

Wet Socks Against Insomnia

A study into the factors that cause insomnia could not come up with a single condition that helped people fall asleep—except for one: cold feet invariably were linked to sleeplessness. Wet socks, therefore, are a powerful nonchemical sleeping aid. As unlikely as it sounds, you will sleep better with wet socks on your feet. The cold, wet socks give a stimulus to rush blood into the feet. After a few minutes, your feet turn warm. Amazingly, Sebastian Kneipp came up with the ridiculous idea of wet socks more than a century before the study confirmed the link between cold feet and tossing and turning in bed.

At bedtime, put on a pair of cotton socks that you have dunked in cold water and wrung out lightly. Pull a pair of dry woolen socks over the wet socks, wrap your feet in a towel, and go to bed. Take the socks off if you wake up in the night. But it's fine to leave them on all night. You will sleep like a baby.

Dry Brushing of the Skin

Brush your dry skin vigorously toward the heart for several minutes with a soft brush or a soft loofah cloth. Start at your feet, and work up slowly in long brushstrokes. Brush your abdomen clockwise (the direction in which the large bowel empties). You can reach your back with a long handle, or ask your partner. Omit your face, nipples, and genital area. Take a bath or a shower afterward.

Dry brushing has many benefits:

- It is invigorating. Not as much as a cold shower and cold washing, but this is a reasonable alternative when water is not available—like in the desert—or temporarily not allowed, as when you are sick.
- It increases circulation to the skin.
- It improves lymph flow.
- It detoxifies the body.
- It helps asthma.
- It increases circulation deep inside the body.
- It exfoliates the skin (removes dead skin cells).
- It fights cellulite.
- It normalizes the production of skin oil.
- It tones and invigorates the whole body.

CAUTION: Do not use this treatment if you have:

- Skin conditions such as psoriasis and eczema
- Too low blood pressure (because it makes it worse)

Walking Barefoot

People have been walking barefoot since the beginning of time. Sebastian Kneipp, who grew up as a poor weaver's son, walked barefoot in spring, summer, and fall out of necessity and discovered the health benefits of walking barefoot when he was forced to wear shoes. He took every occasion to slip out of them. So strip off your shoes and socks, and walk barefoot—at the beach, meandering in and out of the ocean, at a shallow or a little creek, at the shore of a lake—wherever you find cold water. You can walk barefoot in the dewy morning grass or on wet pebbles or happily in the rain in your backyard. You can even walk barefoot in the snow, but only for a very short time—less than a minute. (Stop when your feet hurt.)

Walking barefoot is a relief for the bones and tissue of your feet. It also invigorates your immune system and reduces the frequency of colds and headaches. It is good for treating constipation and prevents or alleviates varicose veins and hemorrhoids.

CAUTION: Do not use this treatment if you have:

- Raynaud's
- Hardening of the arteries in your legs
- An acute urinary tract infection
- Acute lower-back pain

Alternating Hot and Cold Compresses for Treating Injury

The cold of a cold compress reduces swelling and pain by clamping down the vessels. But without blood supply, the site cannot heal. The heat of a hot compress will bring blood back into the area, promoting healing, but will also increase swelling and pain. By alternating cold and hot compresses (fifteen minutes cold, forty-five minutes hot), you get the best of both worlds.

Place an ice pack on the sore area. Keep it in place with a towel, if necessary. After fifteen minutes, replace it with a warm to hot compress: Dunk a kitchen towel in hot water, and apply it as soon as you can stand the heat, or use an electric heating pad or heat a microwavable beanbag (usual heating time is two minutes at high power). Leave the heat on for forty-five minutes (or until it hurts).

This practice soothes acute pain after a bruise or a sprain or acute back pain. It reduces swelling, promotes healing, relieves muscle spasms, increases range of motion in a joint, repairs bruised tissue, and helps in mending bones.

CAUTION: Do not use this treatment if you have:

- Open wounds
- An acute arthritis flare

Cold Wrappings

Most often, cold wrappings are applied on the calves of children to lower fever. Water evaporation from the cloth cools the calves and brings down the fever. In Europe, cold clay wrappings (which prolong cold exposure) are used for treating acute phlebitis and aching varicose veins, but the healing clay can be hard to find elsewhere.

Place a rubber cloth or a plastic bag under the calves. Moisten two clean, soft kitchen towels with cold water from the tap (do not use ice water), wring them out loosely, and wrap them around the calves so that they thoroughly touch the skin, but not too tightly. Do not cover the towels. The wraps reach body temperature in about ten to fifteen minutes and then need to be renewed. Renew not more than twice in one session, and don't apply this more than twice a day without consulting with a physician. Clay wrappings keep the cold longer, about thirty to forty-five minutes.

Always check the color of the toes before you wrap the calves. Are they pink? Apply cold wrappings only on warm, pink limbs.

CAUTION: Do not use this treatment if you have:

- A fever of more than 104°F (consult your doctor at once!)
- Cold hands or feet or pale skin—all signs of centralization—because cold wrappings would clamp down the circulation further

---

Chest Wrapping to Treat Infection, Respiratory Diseases, or Agitation

The use of chest wrappings blocks heat, thus mildly increasing the body temperature. It also loosens bronchial secretions and eliminates waste and toxic substances. It induces sweat and modulates the autonomic nervous system from activity mode to relaxing mode.

First spread a blanket over a bed. Over this, lay a cotton sheet and then a towel across where the patient's chest will be. Over this place a spring cold (32°F to 57°F; 0°C to 14°C), wrung-out cloth folded as wide as the distance from the patient's armpits to his or her navel. Have the patient lie down on this, with arms overhead. Wrap the cloth around him or her tightly (no air pockets), but not tight enough to hinder breathing. Cover the moist cloth loosely with the towel, and then allow the arms to come down next to the body. Envelop the patient now with the cotton sheet, and finally fold the blanket over the patient so that he or she is bundled from head to toe except the face. Leave the patient in this wrap for forty-five minutes. Dim the lights and/or play soothing music. But do not let the patient be unobserved.

The wetter the cloth, the greater the stimulus. Make sure the patient is warm before the procedure; warm him or her first if necessary.

You expect the patient to lightly sweat, look rosy, and feel comfortable within a few minutes. Stop immediately if the patient has a very red face, shortness of breath, complaints about still being cold after five to ten minutes, anxiety, or paleness. Ask the patient frequently whether he or she still feels comfortable. Even if the patient does not voice a complaint, if he or she seems to be uncomfortable, the procedure should be terminated.

Create a quiet environment: no talking, no TV, no radio, no rushing through the room.

Usually this is used for a *Kur* (cure) of about ten chest wrappings, two per week. A single procedure might be sufficient for acute bronchitis to loosen secretions. For inducing sweating during a common cold or the flu—but only if there is already fever—the wrapping can be prolonged to one to two hours. Observe the sick person closely, and determine when the purpose—profuse sweating—has been reached; then finish the session.

CAUTION: Do not use this treatment if the patient has:

- High fever
- Claustrophobia or high anxiety levels
- Acute shortness of breath
- Hyperthyroidism
- Open skin sores in the covered area

Gentle Warm-Water Enema

Enemas gently help evacuation of waste material from the end of the large intestine. They are useful in acute and chronic constipation, and they help with detoxifying during a fast. I do not recommend high colonics—just a gentle warm-water enema. Enemas can be used to retrain the bowel and provide instant, gentle relief of constipation without addictive laxatives. For detoxifying during a fast, they should be done twice a day as long as the fasting continues.

Enemas are not a cure-all. Especially, they do not substitute for healthy nutrition, regular exercise, and good bathroom habits. Never suppress your urge to defecate; always follow nature's call immediately. One should move one's bowels at least once a day. On every day that you did not have a bowel movement, apply a warm-water enema before you go to bed. (See Chapter 20 for dietary suggestions to relieve constipation.)

For this procedure, you will need a soft rubber bulb with a round point; baby ear syringes work well. Fill the bulb with lukewarm water. Do not add anything to the water. Test the temperature with the back of your hand to be sure the water is comfortable and not too warm. Apply a mild cream to your anal area. Gently insert the tip of the bulb while sitting on the toilet. Slowly advance. This should never hurt. Don't push the tip in against resistance and/or pain; it should glide in very easily. Squeeze in the water. Do not hold very long. Evacuate whatever comes out. It might not be much, but it will enhance your next bowel movement. Wash your anal area and clean the rubber bulb with soap and water, rinsing thoroughly. Any soap residue would be an irritant on your next use.

If you cannot find a rubber bulb, you can also buy a commercial enema, discard the contents (they are too harsh), and use the container in the same way.

CAUTION: Do not use this treatment if you have acute hemorrhoids—it would be too painful to insert the tip.

PART 2

MOVEMENT

TO REST IS TO RUST

LIFE IS MOVEMENT. I LEARNED THAT AS A CHILD FROM A story by the German novelist Johann Peter Hebel (1760–1826).

A rich man suffered from so many ailments that no physician had been able to help him. Desperate, he wrote to a famous doctor who lived in a faraway town. The rich man described his symptoms: headaches, exhaustion, cold feet, aches in the joints, belly pains and bloating, shortness of breath, sweating with the slightest effort, loss of joy in life, difficulties with urination and defecation, and more. He requested to visit the famous physician. The doctor answered that the patient was welcome any time; however, the doctor felt that transportation by carriage or on horseback would put the patient at an extreme risk. Namely, the doctor had concluded that the rich man had a rare and easily fatal disease: inadvertently, he must have swallowed a tiny dragon's egg that already had grown huge in his belly, crowding out his organs. Any rough shaking—unavoidable in the carriages of that time—could burst the membranes of the egg, and a dragon with seven jaws would hatch and devour the poor patient from within. There was only one solution: the doctor advised the patient to travel by foot to the faraway town; no other way was known to preserve the dragon's egg and avoid certain death. Once the patient arrived, the doctor would know how to hatch the egg and how to talk to the dragon to make it safely leave the man's body.

So the rich man set out on his long journey. Walking was a bitter task for him, as he was out of the habit. Every night he fell into the bed of another inn, tired and sore in body and mind, often too worn out even to dine. He had no eye for the strange people and interesting trades of the foreign provinces he was passing through. But day by day, his walking became less labored, until he discovered the beautiful valleys, hills, rivers, and forests he walked through. He found the world and the people friendly, and so they found him. Every day, the rich man was up with the sun and on his way, rain or sunshine. He listened to the birds and smelled the flowers in the gardens along the road.

When he arrived at the doctor's office—you guessed it—he was cured from all the ailments and afflictions that had plagued him. He shook the wise doctor's hand and paid him handsomely.

Like this rich man, many of us are carrying "dragon's eggs" in our bellies: the seeds of decline, illness, and early death caused by a lack of movement. Modern life has us sitting in front of computers, standing behind counters, and driving around in cars and trucks. But human beings were made to move on their own feet, not to remain sedentary, and if you rest, you will "rust."

Moving water cleanses itself from impurities. Rivers jumping over rocks sparkle with freshness. Waterfalls fill the air around them with brilliant, thrilling moisture. Standing waters, however, turn muddy, foul, repugnant. Since ancient times, people have known that a stagnant pool breeds disease.

Every cell in your body carries a minuscule pool of water within it and swims in a sea of water outside. And like a river, your body water needs to be stirred and moved to remain clean and fresh, and to delay decay. Eventually, rot, rust, and toxins will get us all—but for now, shake it baby! Moving your body water keeps rot, rust, and toxins at bay, which makes each cell work better individually and all the cells work better together for optimal health.

The Many Benefits of Movement

Once you move from your couch, the positive effects are myriad. For starters, movement cuts your risk of death from heart disease in half. Furthermore, exercise does all these things for you:

- Brings oxygen to your organs, especially your muscles, heart, brain, and kidneys
- Strengthens circulation of the blood through your vessels
- Fights cellulite
- Keeps artery walls flexible
- Increases cardiac output
- Prevents too high and too low blood pressure

- Improves varicose veins
- Averts heart disease and heart attacks
- Postpones aging
- Expands the volume and the health of your lungs
- Builds up muscles
- Curbs cravings and boosts metabolism, helping weight loss
- Fights depression by producing endorphins
- Creates a smarter you by providing more oxygen to the brain
- Deepens sleep at night
- Detoxifies the body
- Gives a glow to your skin
- Works against osteoporosis
- Brings down cholesterol
- Relieves chronic pain
- Reduces stress by breaking down stress hormones faster
- Enhances sexual stamina and exercises sexual muscles
- Improves lymphatic drainage, helping the immune system remove pathogens from your body
- Improves acute and chronic back pain
- Prevents and heals constipation
- Increases the production of acidity in your stomach, which will help you in digestion
- Enhances your overall resistance to infections and diseases

Just a few minutes a day of exercise are enough to give you all of these health benefits. Does that sound too good to be true? Do you think only the big effort at jogging and squash and heavy exercise machines count because they promote the famous cardiovascular health? Well, think again! Too many Americans do not even get a minimum workout because they think a little bit of exercise is not worthwhile. Cave dwellers, our Stone Age ancestors, moved around all day to find food and shelter. But they were just roaming, never jogging!

Turn the page to the next chapter, and discover the two-minute exercise revolution.

CHAPTER 9

GETTING STARTED

THE TWO-MINUTE EXERCISE

REVOLUTION

We are not yet advanced enough to be able to measure the bliss in every one of the billions of cells in your body that comes from even small amounts of exercise. However, you can feel the benefits if you pay attention. With every little movement that you do attentively, you will feel the joy in your body, the feeling of all of those water molecules moving around, the bliss of experiencing a mindful being in a miraculous body. A nice stretch here, a little bend there, a glass of water now and then during the day, a short shake in between tasks—everything adds up so that you feel lighter and more flexible. Your blood will flow more easily, and you will feel the warmth arriving in your fingertips and toes. Done *regularly*, these little movements will build up strength and health.

My ideas about movement and exercise can be summarized in two points:

1. Movement and exercise are absolutely, totally, and unconditionally necessary.
2. Keep it simple and easy: *two minutes a day is enough to begin*.

If you think you can squeeze two minutes into your busy day, read on. We all know how perfect movement looks: beautiful, flowing, elegant, fluid—like a dancer whirling on the stage, like a creek skipping over pebbles. The opposite kind of movement we describe as clumsy, jerky, stilted, inhibited, stiff, and even dead. You want the joy of a sun-dappled brook in your joints, the vigorous flow of a river in your stride, the grace of an overflowing fountain in your spine. And the revolutionary thought is that you can achieve these goals by beginning with just two minutes of exercise a day!

Perhaps you have an old exercise machine—treadmill, bike, stair-climber, elliptical trainer, ski machine, rower—gathering dust in the basement? Clean it up, and pledge to spend just two minutes on it every day. If you do not have access to a machine, you can walk briskly up and down stairs or jump in place. The idea is that you must do it for at least two minutes every single day. If you get carried away and do twenty minutes, that's great, but the next day it is two minutes again! You will begin to notice changes in your body almost immediately, not to mention how proud you'll feel.

Start Moving!

For the sake of clarity, let's divide movements into three kinds. The first mainly involves moving your spine (called micro movements). With the second kind of movement, you do not move your body at all but just tense the muscles and then let go (these are called isometric exercises). And with the third, you add "real" movements of your arms, legs, and whole trunk—normal movements done in sports and gymnastics.

The movements I want to teach you are mainly in the first two categories. For starters, it's better to begin with tiny movements that enable you to listen to your own body than to overexert your muscles. As a physician I know all too well what a toll on the body the infatuation with vigorous sports takes: damaged knees, inflamed tendons, strained muscles—not to mention heart attacks. The whole field of sports medicine stems from people overdoing exercise!

Start with easily doable movements. Be active with your spine, for example, even when you sit or lie. Every time you move the slightest little bit, you relieve stress and tension, and you exercise and strengthen your muscles. Then when you sleep and really do not move much, this extra muscle mass keeps your metabolism burning and makes you lose weight. Muscles at rest burn more than ten times the calories of fat tissue at rest. So every little exercise burns up calories twice—once when you do it and then again at rest when the stronger muscle burns energy at a higher rate than fat. The purpose of fat in the body is to store the most energy with the least amount of energy loss. That is fine in times of starvation, but not in our times of abundant calories. We now die of storing too much fat. So move! Yes, even now while you are reading this book. Wiggle your spine, lift your legs, rotate your shoulders. Lose fat! Build up muscles! And now see how relaxed you feel!

Rather than engaging in these modest forms of movement, many people do not move at all, discouraged that they cannot compete in our "health club" culture. But what is the result? People are not merely overweight now, but morbidly obese, hitting 250 pounds, 300, and more. Obesity, along with its risks of type 2 diabetes, heart disease, and cancer, has become an epidemic. One of the reasons is that people have cut themselves off from what they are feeling inside their bodies. They no longer feel connected to what is going on inside them. I want you to get back into your body and feel it; feel the small, unpretentious, and very precious movements of everyday life.

Ideally, you want to work on muscular strength, muscular endurance, flexibility, and even cardio-respiratory endurance. But don't get too ambitious if you are an exercise novice. Imagine: if you do your two minutes of exercise (or a ten-minute walk) every single day, you are already turning your body from a "couch potato" state to one of greater fitness. Instead of breaking down muscle and bone tissue, your cells suddenly exclaim, "She's using her thighbone!" "He's moving his quadriceps." "Let's build them up again!" By doing your two minutes a day, you begin building a new body, reclaiming your health.

Do any one of the following activities *vigorously and mindfully* for two minutes each day:

- Use any exercise machine: rowing machine, stationary bicycle, elliptical machine, stair-climber, or treadmill.
- Jump up and down in place.
- Run up and down stairs.
- Jump rope.
- Do arm exercises with weights. (Books or water-filled plastic bottles work fine, too.)
- Do one yoga pose. Many books on the market will show you how to do them properly. Of course, a good teacher is best.
- Do push-ups or belly crunches.
- Work with elastic exercise bands. (They come with instructions when you buy them.)
- Install a bar between two doorjambs and do pull-ups.

If You Need a Bigger Challenge

I designed this two-minute beginning exercise program for my patients and myself, and it works very well. But if exercising for two minutes a day isn't enough for you, feel free to design a more rigorous program for yourself or join a professionally run training program. Go for it! Scale the mountains! Make sure, though, that you have a doctor check you out before you start a major workout. And don't hurt yourself: always listen inside!

CHAPTER 10

STAYING MOTIVATED TO MOVE

I t's tough to get motivated to move and to stay motivated, but you can do it! Keep in mind that you need to devote just two minutes a day to exercise, and you'll be on your way to cleansing and detoxifying all the cells and systems in your body—not to mention building a more contented and beautiful self.

If you are new to exercise, here are some tricks for getting started painlessly:

- **Take a cold shower.** A cold shower is a quick way to put your brain into a can-do mode. You may start with a warm or hot shower, as long as you end up with a cold shower. It is an instant mood resetter.
- **Set your goals low.** That seems to fly in the face of everything we've been taught. We set our goals high—very high. Truth is, setting our goals too high has left more than half of the population stranded, exercise-wise, health-wise, and self-esteem-wise. Make your goals realistic or even lower than that, and work your way up; you'll be amazed at how much you can accomplish.
- **Make a plan.** From now on, plan to do two minutes of exercise every single day; the benefits will be amazing. Sticking to your two-minute plan will make you feel proud and accomplished. And you wouldn't believe what two minutes can do for you. For me, two minutes a day on my

ski machine gave me a decent behind for the first time in my life. That's motivation!

- **Tell your friends and family.** To make sure you stay on course, tell people about your new endeavor. Research shows that people stick with their resolutions better if they share the news with friends and family. You could even train with a friend. Perhaps you can start a walking club in your neighborhood and invite people to join.

To get more motivated, consider some of the most common reasons people give to pass on exercise. And then, let's dismantle the excuses. You'll quickly see that some form of exercise can be done by anyone, in any condition.

"I Have No Time"

People say they don't have enough time, but really, even the busiest person can spare two minutes. Just get on your exercise bike, on the treadmill, on the diagonal trainer, on your rowing machine. Work out for two minutes. Do this every single day. It helps to have your machine where you will trip over it: in your office or in front of your TV. In between and all day long, no matter what you are doing, wiggle, fidget in your chair, take the stairs instead of the elevator, park far away from the store, stretch at your desk, do deep breathing whenever you think of it.

Two minutes is not enough, you say? Wrong! Every little bit helps. Research now shows that there is no effort too small that a result can't be seen. The secret is to do it every single day.

"I'm Too Old to Start Now"

Nonsense. More and more studies show that it is never too late to train your muscles. There is no age limitation; people eighty-five and older have done exercises sitting in a wheelchair and enjoyed

KEGEL EXERCISES:
QUICK BUT IMPORTANT EXERCISES FOR WOMEN

Kegel exercises strengthen your "sexual" muscles and will prevent and/or improve pelvic muscle weakness. Done regularly, they help prevent the dreaded organ prolapse and urinary incontinence.

This is the easiest way to learn Kegels: During urinating, try to stop the flow by squeezing your muscles tight. First, nothing much might happen, and you might be unable to stop the flow. After a while, you will succeed and you will learn which muscles to use. Afterward, you can squeeze those muscles tight regardless of where you are. Squeeze them twenty times in a row. Since these are internal muscles, nobody will be the wiser about what you are doing. Once you get stronger, you can introduce variations: squeezing tighter and tighter, squeezing faster and slower, and so on. Kegel exercises take less than a minute to do. You might want to repeat them several times a day.

benefits such as improved strength, mood, balance, and sense of well-being. You don't have to be a sleek goddess or a strapping, muscular hunk. Anybody—*any body*—benefits from movement. Even in your nineties, you can recover some of your lost functions if you are determined. Just go at it slowly, and make sure you're doing the right exercises at the right pace for your body. Always discuss this with your physician.

"I Was Born Unathletic"

In school, I was unathletic; nobody wanted me on their team. Still, that didn't stop me from eliminating the foods that gave me muscle weakness, fatigue, and joint pains and slowly starting to exercise two minutes a day. If I—a premature baby who weighed a little more than four pounds, never thrived, and learned to walk only at age three—could do it, you can do it, too. *Every* body is born for movement; we are not vegetables.

"Too Much Exercise Ruins the Joints"

Movement actually lubricates the joints. Overexercising can ruin your joints, true, and a diet high in inflammatory substances (see the list in Chapter 14) can ruin your joints, but lack of movement is the worst enemy of your joints. *To rest is to rust.*

"There's No Gym near My House"

You don't need a gym next door. Start with hopping on the spot for two minutes, or go for a ten-minute walk. You can work out with a yoga ball, which is relatively inexpensive and versatile, and use it to increase your core abdominal muscles and build overall strength. (See Chapter 12 for suggestions on how to use it.) Try out some exercise machines at stores, gyms, or at your friends' houses. Then buy cheap, used equipment according to your needs. But the truth is, two minutes of any kind of exercise, whether you use a machine or not, will get you started.

Some workplaces offer gyms, classes, and/or athletic games. Make use of them to find out what you enjoy doing. You can also buy audiotapes to guide your workouts at home. I like tai chi, yoga, and breathing, for instance. Videotapes and DVDs can show you what mistakes to avoid, but, if you're a beginner, don't be discouraged by the slim, beautiful, capable instructors doing things that seem impossible to follow. Go at your own pace, and feel good that you're doing it at all!

"Exercise Hurts"

Exercise hurts only if you do it wrong, wear the wrong gear, or overdo it. Watch a cat after she gets up from a nap: She yawns; she stretches; she wiggles in place. Only when she feels comfortable does she consider the next step. We overrule our bodies all the time with our busy brains: have to do this, have to do that.

Exercise, when done right, does not hurt. To the contrary! Studies have shown that mild to moderate exercise dampens pain, probably by distracting the brain and using up nerve paths for pleasurable sensations, and by creating feel-good endorphins. Exercise should feel good in every cell of your body. Give it a try.

"I Can't Compete with . . ."

Exercise should not be about competing. It's about *your* little steps and *your* little effort. In the long run, you might not be satisfied with two minutes a day. I started with two minutes when I was about fifty, but I gradually increased my exercising over time because it felt so good! I know I'll never measure up to movie beauties or professional athletes, but I am healthier, and I am happy in my body now.

Reread the list of benefits of movement at the beginning of the chapters in Part 2. This time, read it out loud—and move! At least wiggle your pinkie!

"Exercise Gear Is So Expensive"

That can be true. But it doesn't have to be. Gear doesn't make you healthy; movement does. I bought a used, old-fashioned cross-country ski machine years ago, cheap. I am still using it. Many people want to get rid of their old machines, so you might find them in a secondhand magazine or online. I also bought a new rower for a little more than two hundred dollars. There are rowing machines for much more money, but they are not necessarily better. I go to yoga class in old sweatpants and a faded sweater. Nobody has complained yet.

"I Can't Afford a Personal Trainer, and on My Own, I Can Never Do It"

I can't afford a personal trainer, and maybe you can't either. But you can be your own trainer. For some ideas, see Chapter 11, which describes exercises for the lazy.

You can also try these other exercise ideas:

- Use books or plastic bottles filled with water as dumbbells.
- Run up and down the stairs for two minutes.
- With your hands, push yourself up on a kitchen counter—or on a shopping cart. But be careful. One time I toppled with the empty cart, landing smack on my belly.
- Follow an exercise or yoga program on the radio, TV, videotape, or DVD. (Try not to look at those impossibly beautiful bodies. Close your eyes, listen to the instructions, and listen to your own body.)

These tricks help me to stick to my exercise plans:

- I have all my exercises on a to-do list. I never do them all in a single day, but it is a joy to check off even one.
- I have a friend who walks with me during lunch hour, and my husband walks with me in the evening.
- Most of all, I am helped when my body reminds me how much better I feel with movement.

"I'm Too Sick to Exercise"

My cat came from the shelter declawed, and in her old age she's turned deaf—stone-deaf. But she still climbs trees and catches mice. Why? I figure because nobody told her that she has no claws or that she is deaf. So she uses what is there.

Unless you are in a coma or are severely injured, there is no health state in which you can't exercise. Movement is possible and useful in all conditions. But you might have to adjust your routine and your expectations. And don't think a few minutes will be too brief to make a difference.

Sometimes, exercise has to be passive, as with physical therapy and quadriplegics. But as Christopher Reeve taught us, bodywork can recover some of the functions that have been lost—at any state. In bed you might be able to wiggle your toes. In a wheel-chair, you can still swing your arms. People with heart failure benefit from moderate walking. Whatever your limitations, always discuss your plans with your physician first.

Some machines, such as an elliptical trainer, require a lot of strength to start with. You might be better off with a rowing machine where you sit comfortably and follow your own pace. Yoga, tai chi, the Feldenkrais Method, or Pilates might be advisable after an injury or with severe restrictions. But again, discuss it with your doctor first. Whatever you do, don't give in to doing nothing, since that will only increase stiffness, deconditioning, pain, and depression. Always remind yourself that every little bit helps!

"Exercise Is Boring"

I, too, find exercise boring—extremely boring. I like to do so many things in life: gardening, reading, practicing medicine, cross-stitching, playing the cello, being with my family and my friends—the list goes on. Exercise is not among them.

But that doesn't keep me from exercising, and it need not stop you. Consider the following tricks to make exercise more interesting:

- Watch your favorite TV show or old movies while on a rowing machine, treadmill, or similar machine. Don't *ever* allow yourself to just sit and gawk at TV without moving your body. But don't train hard while you are not listening to your body—be gentle. Of course it would be better to wholly concentrate on what you are doing. But I admit: I sin here too.
- Read while on a stationary bike. The same cautionary words apply here.
- Change your routine every day or so. Try gardening, alternating machines (rowing, stationary bike, treadmill), walking, hanging out (one of the "lazy exercises" in Chapter 11), and morning bed exercises (also in Chapter 11).
- Change your walking routes. Walk on even ground, in hilly terrain, and on a challenging surface like cobblestones. Change your pace between brisk and leisurely. Walk in an urban setting and also at the beach, in a forest, along fields and meadows. Find out what you like best.
- Walk with a friend (or several). They might pull you out of the house when you want to drop out of the program.
- Get together with a crowd, and play sports. Try volleyball, basketball, soccer, badminton—whatever appeals to you.
- Enroll in an exercise class. Yoga, Pilates, tai chi, and the Feldenkrais Method might appeal to you. Again, companionship might keep you committed.
- Keep a journal. Check off daily what you have done. On my computer calendar, I keep a list of physical activities I might

do—for example, walking, rowing, hanging out, swimming, gardening, neck exercises, bed exercises, jumping on the spot, yoga ball, back exercises, gentle running. I don't do all of them every day—but I do some.

Movement Is Life

Even if you start with only two minutes, you begin to reap all the benefits listed at the beginning of Part 2, because they are cumulative: strength grows on you like money does in the bank. Think of two minutes of daily exercise as saving one dollar per day. It isn't much—but over the years, your account will grow.

If you start with only two minutes a day, soon enough the joy of exercise will have gripped you, and you never will look back to your couch potato days. Your body will crave the feeling of being moved, being exercised, and feeling exuberant.

CHAPTER 11

GO WITH THE FLOW
EXERCISE FOR THE LAZY

I n this chapter, you will find easy, painless ways to begin moving your body with the ease and flow of a brook. The following sequence of stretches and exercises will have you moving before you know it! Do not feel you have to do all of the exercises in this chapter every day. Vary your routine, and pick the ones that your body seems to need on any given day. Listen inside! And don't forget—it's only two minutes! Don't create pressure, create bliss. You will be astonished by how much these simple movements, *done regularly*, will change your body and your mind.

The long-term goal of movement is a combination of endurance (also called cardiovascular fitness), strength, and flexibility. In yoga—which can be regarded as the model for graceful, invigorating exercise—flexibility is the most important element. Strength of your muscles will develop in time, if the postures are done regularly, and the cardiovascular fitness will result from moving faster and more vigorously through the stances. A tiny bit done daily is worth more than a tired muscle, pressed for the umpteenth time. You cannot train a tired muscle, but you surely can damage a tired muscle.

> ### MOVEMENT TIPS TO REMEMBER
>
> - **Movement should be bliss.** If anything starts hurting, back down immediately. Try to do the movement with less force, less often, slower, and with more grace and full attention. It should feel good when you make the right adjustments.
> - **Never lock your elbows or your knees—or even worse, overextend them.** Always hold them with the tiniest, unnoticeable bend.
> - **Never overstretch your back.** Always hold it tight with your buttock muscles.
> - **Drink water before and after exercise.** Movement won't do you any good if it leaves you dry as a prune. It is not necessary to keep a water bottle with you at all times, except during prolonged exercise. Drink lukewarm water. Ice-cold water after exercise might clamp down your heart vessels, setting you up for a heart attack. *And always drink from a beautiful cup.*

Lazy Exercises to Get You Moving

Try these very simple exercises, and you'll discover very quickly how much you gain in health and well-being.

The Stretch of All Stretches: The Diagonal Stretch

1. Sit on a chair with both feet flat on the floor, back and head straight. Lift your right arm. What do you feel?
2. Now do it again. Lift your right arm, but this time press your left foot down onto the ground. Do you feel the movement going straight across your abdomen? Do you feel your spine straightening? Now do the other side!

With the diagonal stretch, you discover your abdominal muscles and the snake in your spine, how it spirals upward, ever so slightly. You feel strength that goes through your whole body. Keep this sensation in mind, because the snake in your back should accompany all your movements. Whenever you are "just" moving an arm or a leg, watch the snake spiral upward, because only then does the movement come from your core—your spine.

What it does: Increases body awareness; strengthens arm, leg, back, and abdominal muscles; improves posture.

Time required: From a few seconds to a few minutes.

Cautions: None.

Micro Movements

"Sit still!" Wasn't that how we grew up? *Don't fidget, don't wiggle. Just sit still.* Our parents were wrong on this point. Studies have shown that people who fidget use up more calories than people who just sit there. And it's not peanuts either; fidgeting uses up quite a chunk of calories. So don't use the remote control; change channels the old-fashioned way, by getting up and walking to the TV.

Do minimal but constant movements throughout your day. Move your hands and feet, your arms and legs. Most of all, move the snake in your spine, and straighten your back! Feel that you are alive at your core. Wiggle! Shake! Move it! I call those snake-like movements *micro movements*. I tell my patients that when I walk into the exam room, I want to see them wiggling in their chairs, instead of just sitting there motionless!

Spinal movements cannot be overemphasized. Move your spine (and the ribs that are attached to it), and all the other parts of your body will get plenty of exercise. This reminds me of a saying I heard from one of my aunts when I was a little girl: Clean the corners, and the middle of the room will be clean without effort.

Feel your spine moving, and the bliss of movement will pervade your whole body.

Spinal movements are barely visible, so there is no competition with anyone. This provides a paradigm shift from competition to bliss. Jogging looks swell when one runs around in a nifty outfit and looks accomplished. But when you move your spine, only you notice your body's joy. And, by the way, your posture will improve, and so will your looks.

You can apply micro movements all day long, while standing, sitting, talking, waiting, but at first they are best learned while lying down on your back.

Micro Movements on the Floor

Getting down on the floor seems like child's play. It is. That is why older folks one day discover that they can't do it anymore. They are out of the habit—and out of flexibility to get down, out of strength to get up. Use it or lose it! So get down daily! Once down, combine it with some fun—with micro movements:

1. Lie flat on your back on a clean carpet, folded blanket, or exercise mat on the floor, arms at your sides. Push down your right arm and shoulder into the floor; now the left. Repeat and be attentive: Do you feel your spine following these movements?
2. Next, forget your arms, and just feel your spine move from side to side. Do you feel the snake hidden in your spine? Make the snake move. Move your shoulders, your pelvis, in a constant, soft flow—but stay flat on the floor. These are micro movements.

Do you feel any pain? If you feel pain in your muscles, just listen to the pain. Move just a bit into the pain. *(Caution: no pushing, no forcing.)* Feel the pain for a moment, then release. If the pain is on the left, move to the right. Do you feel a similar pain here, too? Return to the pain; did it improve? Continue to move from side to side. Play with the pain. Occasionally, you might want to lift your arms up over your head and stretch your back. With arms up, you still can feel the snake move. Imagine you are flying free in the air or floating in supporting waters.

All of these micro movements should be done slowly. Don't exercise—feel! Do micro movements whenever you are idle: sitting, standing, or lying. Keep wiggling all day. In the evening, you will be rewarded with less exhaustion and fewer aches. Micro movements can be combined with deep breathing on awakening, before you even leave your bed (see "Morning Breathing" in Chapter 13). Moreover, they can and should be done whenever you feel unobserved and inactive: in the car (see next exercise), waiting for the bus, doing house chores (preferably with music), reading a book, waiting in line, on a plane, sitting in front of the TV, and so on.

What it does: Increases body awareness; lubricates your joints; straightens your back; improves your posture; builds up muscles and uses up calories.

Time required: There is no extra time required, since micro movements can be done wherever you sit or stand. But if you go down on the floor to do micro movements, allow for a minute or so.

Caution: Don't do this exercise in the car while driving. But you can do it at the red light—be especially careful and observant of your surroundings.

Micro Movements in the Car (for Passengers Only)

Sit with your bottom moved deep into the seat, and start by pushing the top of your head upward as if you want to grow out over the roof of the car or want to push the crown of your head into the heavens. Press back first one shoulder, then the other to awaken the snake in your spine. Pay attention to how the sensation changes every moment.

Find other little movements for your spine, such as rotating the pelvis on the spot, pushing one leg against the floor and releasing, or turning your head slowly. Don't try this at the steering wheel!

What it does: Fights fatigue and the effects of aging; keeps your spine supple; strengthens your back muscles; improves your posture; prevents the usual slumping over in the car; and prevents and remedies back pain.

Time required: Whenever you have a few seconds.

Cautions: Do not do these movements if you have acute back pain. With any pain that is severe or lasting, consult with your doctor.

Arching Your Back

Arching your back is an immediate wake-up call for your spine. You can combine it with micro movements or do it alone whenever you need to realign your posture. Lie down flat on your back. With deep inhaling, push your heels down into the ground, and feel your back and neck straighten into a long, strong line. You might even lift slightly into a long flat arch, suspended by only your heels and shoulders/head. Continue to breathe. Release the posture with an exhale. Repeat twice. If you feel mild pain, notice where it is, and observe how it changes with the gentle movement. If the pain is severe, stop.

While standing, you can get a similar back stretch by clasping your hands behind your back and slowly lifting your arms as high as you can. This pulls back your shoulders, opens your lungs, and releases your back.

Another quick realignment of your spine: hold onto a table or a sink or the hood of your car, step back, and bend horizontally from the hips, with a slight pull backward. (Be careful not to rip the sink out of the wall!) You might hear little cracking noises in your spine while you stretch gently.

What it does: Realigns your spine; straightens your back; and strengthens your leg, back, and buttock muscles.

Time required: One minute tops.

Cautions: Do not do these exercises if you have acute back pain. When doing them, do not overarch your lower spine. Don't get frustrated if initially you cannot lift from the ground. You will develop strength with time.

The Three Laziest Back Exercises

The following suggestions are for people who have back pain but have not started to do anything about it, or for people who want to prevent back pain. About 80 percent of Americans can expect to get at least one episode of debilitating lower-back pain during their lifetimes. If you do not yet have a daily back routine and doubt that you will stick with an elaborate one for long, try these lazy exercises for your back—every single day:

For all three parts, lie flat on the floor on a yoga mat or folded blanket. Place your feet near your buttocks, so that your knees are up, about hip width apart.

1. Lift your buttocks, and fold your hands behind your back. Now roll back and forth from one shoulder to the other, twenty times. Release and relax.
2. Lift your buttocks, and lift your arms up over your head. Again move from one shoulder to the other, twenty times. This feels like fishtailing. Release and relax.

3. Lift your buttocks, arms loosely at your sides. Now circle your pelvis vertically in one direction ten times, then ten times to the other, without touching the floor. Release and relax.

What it does: Strengthens your back muscles; straightens your spine; improves your upright posture; and shapes your behind.

Time required: Less than five minutes.

Cautions: Do not do these exercises if you have acute back pain. Do not overexert yourself initially; start slowly.

Balance

Every time you brush your teeth, stand on one leg, alternating legs. It's that easy!

What it does: Balancing prevents falls. To balance on one leg, you exercise many small and big muscles (including your sexual muscles). Even more important, you exercise your brain and the pathways from your brain to the muscles (the nerves). By balancing daily, you make sure that these systems and pathways do not decline but keep getting more vigorous. And balancing on one leg teaches you that life is about staying upright through difficult times: juggling the needs of work and play, sleep and activity, and your personal-growth needs with the needs of your family and friends.

Time required: Three to five minutes—the time your dentist recommends for toothbrushing (shorter with an electrical brush). At least twice a day.

Caution: Start out by leaning against a support.

Two Minutes on a Ski Machine

I did my first "athletic" exercises on an old NordicTrack machine—two minutes at a time. I could not face the boredom of exercising longer, but I also knew I needed to do something against rusting and sagging. When I saw the miracle effects of two minutes of exercise a day, I advertised the idea to my patients. There was not one who wouldn't say with a grin, "Sure, I can do two minutes!"

What it does: Using a ski machine invigorates and tones the whole body. It also strengthens the muscles of the pelvic floor. That's especially good for women, because it invigorates sexual muscles and works against urinary incontinence and "drooping organs."

Time required: Two minutes.

Cautions: If you have acute joint inflammation of the lower extremities, do not do this exercise. Before engaging in any kind of cardiovascular training (doing this longer than two minutes), consult your physician. Balancing on the skiing machine might be difficult in the beginning. Start with leg movements, while you are holding on tight with your hands. Add arm movements only after you feel safe.

S-l-o-w Motion Weight Lifting

The idea here is to lift weights—using dumbbells, soup cans, water-filled plastic bottles, or books—in very slow motion. Follow these simple steps:

1. Become aware of every little muscle. Do not use heavy weights. In this exercise, more is less.
2. Do not work up a sweat. Try to do every motion with beauty and grace. Think, "How can I lift my arm more

slowly? More elegantly? More softly?" Observe how every movement originates in your trunk and your spine. For instance, when you lift your arm and bend your elbow, concentrate on opening your shoulder and making your armpit wide, instead of focusing on lifting your hands.

3. After you have put the weights down, play with your hands: Stretch out your wrists, stretch out your fingers—even overstretch your fingers a little. Do both arms feel the same? How about one little pinkie?

4. Now return awareness to your armpit: is it still open after you had your attention on your hands? Scan each part of your body: does every part feel open and aligned? Can you still try more softly?

What it does: Builds up body awareness and stamina.

Time required: Two to five minutes.

Cautions: If you have overstressed or damaged joints, do not do these exercises.

Hanging Out

Install a bar securely across a narrow hallway. Pull yourself up ten times. If you cannot lift your feet from the floor, do it anyway— with your feet on the ground. When you are hanging out, your weight will lengthen and straighten your spine. Over time, you will get stronger—and one day you might be able to pull yourself up. Even if not, the exercise lengthens and releases your spine.

What it does: Strengthens arm muscles, straightens your spine, frees intervertebral disks, and improves your posture.

Time required: Less than a minute.

Caution: Make sure the bar is fastened securely.

Morning Bed Exercises

Before you jump out of bed in the morning, do a few very simple stretches: Stretch your arms over your head and wiggle. Turn onto your belly, and push up slightly onto your arms to gently lengthen your back. Gently rotate your neck. Get onto your knees, and curl down into a ball.

What it does: Awakens your spine and your mind.

Time required: Less than a minute.

Caution: Be careful not to overstretch your lower back on a too-soft mattress.

When You Are Ready for More Exercise

In case you become so enthusiastic about movement and exercise that you want to do more, it is important to find out what constitutional type you are and to choose your exercises accordingly. The lighter your build, the lighter the exercises you should take up. Most people are, of course, a mixture between the types. This list provides only suggestions:

- **Light exercises:** yoga, tai chi, swimming, skating, walking, gentle running, bicycling, rowing, skiing (downhill and cross-country), badminton, volleyball, archery, fencing, gymnastics, ballet, dance, golf, horseback riding
- **Medium exercises:** yoga, tai chi, walking, gentler martial arts, shorter hikes, low-impact aerobics, swimming, gentle running, bowling, skiing (downhill and cross-country), fencing, rowing, hockey, baseball, basketball, football, surfing, light weight lifting
- **Heavy exercises:** yoga, tai chi, heavier martial arts, walking and all sports where competition comes into play, including

tennis, most ball games (probably not basketball), heavy
weight lifting, surfing, skiing (downhill and cross-country),
gentle running, rowing

Movement should be a part of your life every day, every waking minute. If you want to expand on the exercises in this chapter
and are interested in yoga, tai chi, or other practices, choose an
audiocassette that you can follow every morning. Morning is the
best time of the day for movement, because you open up your
lungs, your joints, your heart, and your brain to the new day and
get a good foundation to handle the day's inevitable stresses. In
the evening, you can do more calming exercises and meditation.
But whatever you choose, make sure you don't forget to wiggle
each and every day.

CHAPTER 12

PERFECT POSTURE
MOVING WITH THE FLOW OF WATER

Imagine a queen or a king entering a room. What is different from how *you* would enter? And why is there a difference? There should be none. But a perfect posture is very hard to maintain. It does not come naturally for most of us. Why not? Because our upright position has developed only in the last million years or so—a blink of an eye in evolution—our bodies still need to be educated. And like water flowing down a mountain, we must acknowledge and work with the pull of gravity.

We all would have perfect spinal alignment and no back problems if we would still walk on all four extremities the way our closest relatives, the apes, do. Ever since we decided to stand up to get a better look out over the savanna to spot food and enemies, we have had the delicate task of balancing our top-heavy head on our swaying spine and two small feet. From there stem all of our problems with posture. Bad posture can cause headaches, back pain, fatigue, and eventually a permanently distorted, bent back.

The secret to perfect posture lies in regular micro movements: your bones need to be wiggled into better alignment constantly. If your bones are in perfect alignment, then you have perfect posture. It is relatively easy to have perfect posture when you are lying down. But as soon as you get up in a sitting or standing position, something happens to this bag of bones that is your body: gravity pulls you—and all of your body water—down.

The spine can be held upright only when the muscles are strong enough to keep it upright. The solution to addressing bad posture (and back pain, neck pain, headaches, and knee or hip pain) is not a better bed or a waist belt or a back brace. You need to create your own internal "scaffolding" through practice and strengthening.

Tips for Perfect Posture

When trying to strengthen and straighten out your spine, follow these simple tips:

- **Move constantly.** Walk on the spot, shift weight from one foot to the other, never stand stock-still. Apply what you learned from micro movements (see Chapter 11) to your standing position. If you must stand still, stand evenly on both feet. Having all your weight on one leg alone can start a lopsided posture. If you must stand for a prolonged time, put one foot higher than the other—on a crate or a step— while keeping your weight evenly distributed. Change sides frequently. This releases tension in your lower back.
- **Become self-aware by watching yourself in a mirror.** Ask yourself about your posture: Am I straight? Is my head tilted? Do I look rigid or natural? Is my butt tucked under? Are my knees and elbows slightly soft? Is my lower spine too flat? Too curved? Are my shoulders at the same height?
- **For prolonged sitting, have a chair that promotes good posture.** A kneeling chair—which allows you to kneel instead of sit—is a good solution in front of the computer. So is a yoga ball or a balance cushion; both promote active sitting instead of passive slumping. I wrote this book in a recliner with a board across for my laptop. I wiggle in place (which improves thinking, too!). And I get up frequently to

do little exercises. Another way to keep good posture while sitting (including in the car) is to place a pillow behind your lower back (lumbar area). But beware of overarching your lumbar area; always listen to your body by listening to any new pain.

- **When sitting, wiggle your sitting bones against the chair until you're sitting perfectly straight.** Never cross your legs when sitting. It leads to varicose veins and puts lopsided pressure on your spine. Have a little footstool handy. To avoid slumping, sit on the edge of your chair and stretch out one foot while keeping the other closer to you. Don't lean on the table; that ruins perfect posture.

- **Sleep on a firm mattress.** Most people choose too soft a mattress. Your pillow should not be too high or too low; your neck spine should not tilt up or down; level is perfect.

- **Sleep with a pillow between your knees.** This brings your spine into alignment and also prevents the dreaded sleeping wrinkles.

- **Use a massage chair.** It's an incredible luxury, especially after a hard day's work. I once used one at a friend's house. It was bliss!

- **Get down on the floor often, and arch your back.** Do this at least once a day. For more details about this stretch, see "Arching Your Back," one of the lazy exercises in Chapter 11.

- **Enroll in a yoga class, or explore other forms of movement education.** When you finally learn natural alignment the way yoga teaches, your back will never be the same. For back pain, Trager movement education, a neuromuscular therapy, helps; it is also very helpful in neuromuscular diseases like Parkinson's. Another excellent way to improve posture is the Feldenkrais Method, a technique that involves thinking, sensing, moving, and imagining. Alexander Technique frees you from habitual, injurious movement patterns.

CAUTION: Be careful not to practice wrong movements. Get your initial instructions from a good physical therapist or a movement teacher. Do not force your new posture. This will be a lifelong process; there will always be room for further improvement.

Three Simple Exercises for Perfect Posture

Here are three easy techniques for helping you develop a straight spine. Remember, as water flows down a mountain, you must work with the pull of gravity.

Developing Perfect Posture

1. Straighten your lumbar area by tucking in your butt and lifting your spine from the waist up. Let your head grow

---

HEALTH CONDITIONS THAT MAY AFFECT YOUR POSTURE

Various health conditions may have an effect on the positioning of your spine, so take particular care if you suffer from any of these problems:

- Obesity
- Pregnancy
- Shoes with high heels (or bad-fitting shoes generally)
- Flat feet or other foot problems
- Fear, anxiety
- Food allergies and intolerances
- Muscle, neurological, and metabolic diseases
- Insufficient sleep

into the heavens by straightening your neck. Do not lift
your chin; do not drop your chin.

2. Relax your shoulders by rolling them down and outward.
   Let go of your shoulder blades. Keep your knees and elbows
   always a tiniest bit bent.

3. Think of growing imperceptibly and infinitely out from the
   two ends of your spine: down from the lumbar area, and up
   from the waist, all the way into the neck. Feel the strength
   of your back; feel your strength. Smile!

4. Do not just sit, lie, or stand there: reposition yourself often.
   For evolutionary reasons, the upright posture is so alien to
   us that we have to regain it a thousand times over the course
   of a day. Good posture depends on a good memory. The
   more often you remind yourself, the better your posture
   will be.

5. Do not squeeze your shoulders together, and do not pull
   them up. Although that is called good posture, military
   style, it is not what you need.

6. Do not bend your head backward. The movement always
   comes from your spine, not from rolling your head around.
   Your head just balances delicately on top of the heap of
   bones and muscles that are you.

What it does: Slowly this exercise will improve your posture
and your mood by strengthening the right muscles and bringing
the many spinal joints in alignment.

Time required: There is no extra time involved; you do
it whenever you notice slumping—for instance, now! In the
beginning, you might do this only once or twice a day and then
forget about it. Later, as your body awareness grows, slouch will
alarm your body immediately into correcting your posture. Initially,
you might feel too lazy to change your posture (for instance, in
front of a TV), and you might have to admonish yourself. But as you
experience the benefits of better posture—even if only for seconds
at first—your body will seek the feeling of bliss.

Props needed: None.

Cautions: None.

The following two exercises will help you develop better posture, but they need some props. Both can be done without the props but are so much easier to accomplish with them.

Headstand

A headstand is an inversion exercise. Imagine reversing the flow of a waterfall inside your body. For doing an easier headstand, you will need a prop called a BodyLift, a small stool-like contraption with an opening for your head. With the BodyLift, your weight rests on your shoulders, sparing the weak neck and spine. You can order a BodyLift or a similar device from specialty stores, a mail-order catalog, or the Internet. I would go for the least expensive brand.

1. Place the BodyLift prop close to a wall.
2. Kneel in front of the prop, facing the wall and holding the front legs of the BodyLift with your hands. Place your head and neck into the opening. Wiggle your shoulders flat onto the padding.
3. Slowly stretch out your legs and walk them up to your body as close as it feels comfortable. Then raise your feet to the upright, inverted position. Your weight rests on your shoulders, and you are still holding on to the front legs of the BodyLift with your hands.
4. If you have never done this, use the wall for support. Even better, let someone hold your feet. It is amazingly easy to do the headstand with this prop, but initial help is safer.

What it does: The headstand, like all the inversion positions, counteracts the sagging force of aging. These positions carry more nourishing blood to the brain and to less used parts of your body—for instance, to the upper lungs. The BodyLift prop makes headstands perfectly easy to do without any neck strain and the anxiety that comes with it. Since all your weight is resting on your shoulders, your head is hanging freely, which will free your neck bones from the constant burden of balancing the heavy head.

Time required: I recommend beginning with one minute and then working up to your desired time minute by minute until you reach five to ten minutes.

Props needed: BodyLift device.

Caution: If you are not in at least moderate condition, use the BodyLift device under the guidance of a yoga teacher or physical therapist. Do not use this treatment if you have:

- Uncontrolled high blood pressure
- Glaucoma
- Pregnancy
- Balance problems (for example, vertigo)
- Neurological difficulties

Back Bend over a Yoga Ball

To do these back bends, you will need a large, inflatable yoga ball that allows you to lie with your upper shoulders and head comfortably on the ball while your feet are flat on the floor. (Yoga balls come in different sizes.)

1. Place your feet on the floor, and lie backward onto the ball so that your upper shoulders and your head rest comfortably on the ball.
2. Slowly and deliberately roll your head, shoulders, and neck back and forth over the ball. Do not lose contact between the ball and the back of your head, but over time, try to increase the amount by which you bend back.

What it does: Increases flexibility of your spine, decreasing a hunch. Also increases muscle strength in your legs, back, and abdomen.

Time required: From one minute upward.

Props needed: Yoga ball. You can buy one from a specialty store, a mail-order catalog, or the Internet. It can be used for all kinds of fun gymnastic games (your ball will likely come with a description of some of these). Some people even use the ball at their desk instead of a chair—for active sitting. It keeps the legs engaged and active and promotes the corrective spinal wiggling that I recommend.

Caution: Do not let your head dangle in the air; maintain contact with the ball at all times. Keep your feet on the floor to not lose balance. Do not do it if you are balance-impaired for any reason.

CHAPTER 13

BREATHING

YOUR MOST IMPORTANT MOVEMENT

Breathing is moving—and it's life's most critical movement. When you are breathing, your respiratory muscles pull your chest wall up and gravity brings it down again. Without this constant moving of your rib cage, brought forth by your chest muscles, you would be dead. You could have perfectly healthy lungs, but if your chest wall is not moving, you will die (that is why children afflicted with polio were put into the iron lung in the fifties). Your lungs provide oxygen, and your heart pumps the oxygen into every tiny vessel of your body. Your heart started beating long before you were born, when you were a tiny embryo just a few weeks old, and has not stopped since. Your heart is nothing more than a big muscle pouch, divided into four chambers by muscle walls, and it contracts once every second or so, even when you sleep.

So whether you are consciously aware of it or not, your body is moving all the time. The brain takes the biggest chunk of oxygen provided by this heart-lung interaction, but all the other organs demand their share, too—the kidneys, the muscles (even when you are not doing much, they still need oxygen), the liver, and the lungs and the heart themselves, just to mention a few.

If you do nothing else suggested in this book but the cold-water shower and the breathing exercises in this chapter, you will make significant changes in your life and health.

You might think you don't need breathing exercises because you breathe all the time anyway! Yes, but unfortunately most people use far less than 50 percent of their breathing capacity—more like 20 percent, in fact. Our breaths are so shallow that they barely deliver enough of the precious oxygen to all of our organs. Breathing is free. It is there for the taking. Breathing deeply does not use up any more time than shallow breathing; all you have to do is remind yourself and get that extra oxygen boost into your system.

Some Oxygen Enriching Breathing Exercises

Use these exercises to nourish your body with oxygen.

Basic Breathing

1. Always start with breathing out. Only a deep exhalation empties your lungs enough to make them open for your next deep inhalation. And always breathe deeply into and out of your abdomen, rather than your chest. (Abdominal breathing is a yoga technique. Put your hand on your navel and feel how your breath moves your belly!)
2. Inhale and count while you inhale. Exhale and count while you exhale. Make sure that your exhaling lasts longer than your inhaling. It does not matter how fast you count as long as you count exhalation and inhalation at the same speed. Count at your own personal pace.
3. Do not hold your breath at the two reversing points between exhaling-inhaling and inhaling-exhaling. Instead, just let the change happen as imperceptibly and smoothly as the tides turn, from ebb to flow, from high to low.

What it does: The breath is your link to life, so improve your life by breathing better. Inhale oxygen; exhale carbon dioxide.

In yoga tradition, you are breathing in more than oxygen, you breathe in *prana*—the life force.

Time required: This exercise requires no extra time; you just have to think of it. Start with reminding yourself every hour on the hour—while awake—to take three deep breaths. Make it a lifelong habit. Why not try it right now? Always begin with breathing out. Always breathe through your nose.

Props needed: None.

Caution: Always breathe through your nose. Do not breathe too fast. If you tend to hyperventilate, stick to the rule that exhalation has to be longer than inhalation.

Morning Breathing

When your alarm rings, stay in bed. Don't jump out of your bed, starting your day in an unhealthy fashion. Instead, breathe in what the Indian yogis call *prana*: the energy that is life.

1. Turn on your stomach with your arms stretched over your head, your legs stretched out, and your face to either side or down—whatever you prefer. Breathe seven times slowly and deeply out and in through your nose. Stretch your back when you breathe in. Don't force the breath.
2. Turn on your back with your legs stretched out and your arms stretched out over your head. Breathe seven times slowly out and in without forcing the breath. Now place your arms loosely at your sides, and breathe another seven times in the same way.

What it does: You may have to try it to believe it, but at this point, you really want to get out of bed because so much energy has entered your body through *pranayama*, yoga breathing.

Time required: Less than five minutes.

Props needed: None.

Caution: Never hold your breath. Make your breath a continuous flow out and in.

Fast Evening Breathing

The evening breathing has to be different from the morning breathing because it should not pump up all your energies to get you out of bed. It should relax you.

1. Open the window before you go to bed.
2. Lie either on your back or in your final snugly sleeping position. Breathe fast back and forth through your nose with a pumping noise. Start at a slower pace until you get a regular rhythm, then slowly speed up your breathing. Never open your mouth. If you run out of breath (which will happen until you get the hang of it), stop the nose breathing and take a slow, deep breath. Then resume the fast nose breathing.

What it does: Relaxes you. Because of its fast pace, this seems to be an exciting exercise. But you will notice afterward that it has taken all stress and tension away.

Time required: Less than two minutes.

Props needed: None.

Caution: Do not hold the breath; make it flow.

Five-Minute Meditation

Meditation embraces the paradigm of merely being or nondoing (also of nonhaving). Doing and having are very much overemphasized in Western culture. Meditation brings you back into your *being* mode whenever you feel overwhelmed and distraught, preferably before you are locked too much into having and doing.

Choose a quiet corner. Put your egg timer on five minutes. Find a sitting position that you can keep for five minutes. You can sit cross-legged on a cushion on the floor or you might choose a chair with a back. Keep your back straight. Do not move at all except to keep your back straight. Hold your hands on your knees, with your palms up and open.

Close your eyes, and breathe in and out slowly without holding or forcing. Just observe your breath. If your thoughts stray, gently bring them back to your breathing. Don't berate yourself for not getting the meditation right—there is no right or wrong, just being and benign observation.

Stop when the clock rings. Go on with your day, enjoying your renewed energy and purpose.

What it does: Meditation calms brain waves, thereby staving off aging of the brain. Meditation helps with concentration and attention span, and increases contentment. It calms you and focuses your mind on your inside. This is a good exercise for the fall, when depression and seasonal affective disorder are triggered by lower light, and introspection is in order. It can help with smoking cessation. Meditation also might help in alleviating the following symptoms:

- Anxiety and panic attacks
- Boredom and procrastination
- Chronic pain

- Fatigue
- Food binges
- Headaches
- High blood pressure
- Insomnia
- Lung diseases
- Mild depression
- Premenstrual syndrome (PMS)
- Stress

Time required: Five minutes. Meditation is ideal in the morning, right after you get up—a wonderful way to greet the day—and in the evening before retiring. It can also be done in your car (after you have parked!) between coming from work and rushing into your house for the evening chores: Shut off the motor, and take those five minutes for yourself. You will notice how those five minutes melt tensions away.

Props needed: Egg timer.

Caution: Don't go longer than five minutes without guidance of an experienced meditator as prolonged meditation could bring out anxieties. If you feel that your depression is worsening with this exercise, consult a physician.

PART 3

FRESH FOOD

BURSTING WITH WATER
AND FLAVOR, GIVING LIFE

MY CAT, A RED TABBY FROM A SHELTER, ARRIVED IN OUR home with some quirks from her former life, including a flat refusal to eat anything but canned cat food. Then one day, she developed a bad eye infection. We spent a lot of time and money at the veterinarian and on medication, but nothing helped. When the infection took over the other eye and she seemed to be going blind, I asked myself what I would do with her if she were one of my human patients and had an incurable disease. Of course, I would apply the Five Water Essentials to strengthen her immune system. Since she gets plenty of exercise (she is an outdoor cat), drinks fresh water, and is—like all cats—a model for a balanced lifestyle without stress, only nutrition and herbs were left for me to tinker with.

I changed her diet to raw beef and raw chicken liver, with the occasional teaspoon of canned food. Initially, she was quite upset with me. But within a week, her eyes began healing. She has had several relapses whenever she eats too much canned food, but she always heals again when on a good diet. Lately I observe that she herself prefers fresh food over canned. Raw liver might not be your idea of gourmet eating. But it is—for a cat. Cats in the wild eat raw meat. What would humans in the wild eat? Fresh food, of course.

CHAPTER 14

HEALTH-BY-WATER NUTRITION
FRESHNESS IS EVERYTHING!

Foods are the building blocks of your body. You don't want to build your body from crummy, poor quality material. And yet most people eat poorly in this country that is supposedly the richest in the world. To make up for poor food choices, they pop a few vitamins afterward. But health cannot be bought from shelves and in bottles.

There was a time when scientists thought life's essentials were the three macronutrients—protein, fat, and carbohydrates. Then they discovered some essential micronutrients: minerals and vitamins (literally, *vital amines*). These discoveries enabled them to invent food with a long shelf life, "improved" with added vitamins and other micronutrients. But since we started to live on fortified cereals, enriched breads, fruit-flavored bars and pastries, and enhanced, pasteurized dairy products, our health has become worse than ever because such manufactured food cannot substitute for the real fresh stuff.

Fresh, Natural Food Is Everything

Food can make you well, or it can make you sick. Some old healing traditions have known this for thousands of years: Tibetan medicine, ayurvedic medicine, or Traditional Chinese Medicine—they all view food as vital to health. European Natural Medicine (ENM) is not as old as the other healing traditions, but growing up in Germany in the traditions of ENM I learned early on: food choices are health choices. Western medicine has long neglected the healing aspect of food—just look at what hospitals dish up to their patients. Now, with the epidemic of obesity in this country, conventional physicians are scrambling to find a cure. But still they overlook what old traditions have long known: health comes from *fresh* food—from a succulent apple for instance, bursting with moist vitality that becomes your own—confirming the billions-of-years-old cycle of life.

Only fresh foods, bursting with life-giving water, will give you the victory of good health and will vanquish disease. Freshness means that the water inside the cells of the food is not rotten, that the enzymes and vitamins have not yet disintegrated, the oil has not turned rancid, and the starch has not become musty. Forget for now calories, carbohydrates, fats, and proteins, vitamins, and other supplements! The one thing you really have to know about nutrition is: freshness.

Keep It Simple, Whole, and Fresh

Prepare your meals from fresh (living) ingredients, preferably organic. Eat mostly whole foods, and avoid processed foods. Stick with easy self-made dishes instead of elaborate courses (save those for festive days), so you taste the real food—a vegetable bursting with water, lentils, brown rice—a simple but delicious meal! Reeducate your taste buds. How does a fresh potato taste without any topping (save, perhaps, a sprinkle of salt or fresh chives)? How about some peas, fresh from the garden, succulent and scrumptious, peeled by hand, and eaten raw as a snack?

Good food is fresh, bursting with vital ingredients, varied, and preferably organic and should be eaten in moderation. It has no shelf life and tastes good without the addition of sugar and salt and artificial flavorings. Good food is good not because it is the "moral" way to eat or because it is popular, but because it matches our ancient physiology. Fancy new molecules like fat or sugar substitutes, dyes, artificial flavors, colorings, and preservatives confuse and poison our old-fashioned bodies—not to mention pesticides, herbicides, antibiotics, hormones, plastics, or whatever else finds its way into our food.

One rule of thumb: do not buy food that is advertised on TV. Have carrots or kale ever been advertised on TV? Advertisements help sell foods with a long shelf life only. Learn to equate long shelf life with inferior food, dead matter, lack of vitality.

Poor nutrition is one of the largest avoidable risk factors for cancer. We already heard that artificial molecules and stale products are bad—right up there with smoking and alcohol abuse. Fresh food is not rancid, moldy, shrunken, shriveled, smelly, or cardboardy. It is not processed, enriched, enhanced, improved, or adulterated in any way. Fresh food is alive with water and vigor. Fresh food is also not coated, painted, or beautified. It does not remind you of plastic. Fresh food is naturally colorful, like in red beets, green kale, yellow summer squash—not because it has been treated with yellow dye #5. But fresh food is also just what it is—spots and all—as it has grown at its own pace, in its own time and season, and in its own healthy soil. Fresh food is not sprayed or irradiated or artificially fertilized or gene manipulated or injected with hormones. Fresh food is, by definition, whole and organic. Whereas modern food manufacturing has taken the freshness and flavor out of food in favor of perfect looks and a long shelf life instead.

A Healthy Body Is Built from Healthful Food Choices

The laws of nature apply everywhere—even to you and me. If we eat pizza and doughnuts, we will build a pizza-and-donut body. Here are some facts you need to consider when choosing your foods:

- Manufacturers do not have your health at heart. Their profit is the bottom line.
- The federal Food and Drug Administration (FDA) does not have your health at heart. The new food pyramid still recommends dairy and milled flour and allows refined sugars, all of which have been shown in studies to have negative health consequences.
- Sadly, most physicians, nutritionists, and dietitians are not aware of the latest scientific information on wholesome food choices.
- Even many so-called alternative-medicine doctors are peddling supplements, from which they make a profit, more than in good health. But a dead pill or a powder cannot bestow life to you. Be suspicious of any nutritional "adviser" who wants to sell you something—whether it is a vitamin, mineral, supplement, food product, or "miracle" diet.

The Health-by-Water Freshness Pyramid

In my years of medical practice, I developed an altogether new food pyramid, which I call the Freshness Pyramid. My Freshness Pyramid is based on foods that are both closest to their natural origins and often have the highest water content. By this measurement, an apple is fresher than home-cooked applesauce, which is fresher than apple pie, which is fresher than an apple-flavored nutrition bar. Likewise, edamame (soybeans still in their pods, cooked to a tender green) is fresher than tempeh (a traditional fermented soy food), which is fresher than soy milk, which is fresher than tofu (a highly processed soy food—nothing in nature comes in a square form), which is fresher than a tofu burger. Milk directly from the udder of a cow is fresher than farm-made cheese from unpasteurized milk, which is fresher than a plain full-fat yogurt, which is fresher than homogenized, pasteurized, growth-hormone-laced skim milk, which is fresher than a yogurt with fruit aroma. A piece of grass-fed lamb is fresher than a corn-fed steak, which is fresher than a salami, which is fresher than canned breakfast meat. A European-style whole-grain heavy sourdough bread is fresher than a soft loaf of so-called whole wheat bread, which is fresher than a Wonder bread of highly milled flour, which is fresher than saltines with their endless shelf life. I think you get the idea: the less food is processed and removed from its original source, and the shorter its shelf life, the better it is for your health.

The Stone Age Diet: An Ideal Model

After we have established freshness as the most important feature of food, now we come to ask: What to eat? What food is natural to us? A cave dweller's diet is natural to us because that's where we came from. Their hunters' and gatherers' fare was varied through the seasons, and it was mostly but not totally vegetarian; now and then, a mammoth had to be devoured. Or some grubs. And they drank water, not soda or sports drinks or fortified juices. For millions of years, the conditions of what and how humans' ancestors ate did not change much, and our physiology is adapted to those ancient conditions. Our forefathers could not afford to be choosy, because starvation was always a threat. That we still celebrate the winter solstice with a great feast and candlelight and spring with all sorts of festivities has to do with how dangerous the cold and dark time of the year was for our ancestors: not everybody made it through into the new growing season.

Aside from freshness, Stone Age nutrition can teach us three things:

1. **Eat varied.** Cave dwellers' diets changed through the seasons and with the different habitats they roamed. They did not eat the same thing day in, day out.

2. **Eat individually.** There never was *the* cave dweller. Stone Age individuals inhabited different climates, different continents, different landscapes; even two adjacent valleys would have provided different food supplies. And each one of us modern descendents contains elements of this varied heritage, whirled about and mixed up by constant migrations, thrown in to create each person's own individuality. The end product is not predictable and a single diet prescription does not fit everybody and every body.

3. **Have a fast once in a while.** Cave dwellers were often challenged by low provisions, and studies have shown that undereating, at least once in a while, prolongs life span in mice and men.

Healthful Food Comes from Healthy Soil

People complain about bland tomatoes from the supermarket, cardboard vegetables, and meat that smells odd when you fry it in the pan. Once I ate a simple salad in one of those little taverns in the Greek countryside. It was just tomatoes, cucumber, onions, and a little olive oil—nothing more, not even salt. But, ah, what a taste, what an unforgettable, delicious taste! Why? Because the soil had not been depleted of nutrients by chemical fertilizers, because it was not polluted by pesticides and herbicides, because the produce was grown close to where it was harvested (in the backyard) and had ripened on the vine or tree or bush. The last few years have seen a resurgence of organic foods, even in conventional supermarkets. As more people are asking for better nutrition, organic has gone mainstream. But the best still grows in your backyard or comes from the local farmers' market.

Why Fresh, Organic Food Is Better for You

Common sense and natural instinct will tell you what is fresh. The more processing steps your food has gone through, the less fresh it is. And it doesn't stay fresh just because you bought it fresh. If you just let your produce linger in your fridge, it gets old and stale because fresh food is still alive (to a degree). And because it is living, it is prone to decay and rot. During transport, in the store, and in your fridge, your fruits and vegetables lose taste and healthful ingredients.

Fresh food includes all produce (fruit and vegetables), nuts, grains, legumes (beans, lentils, peas, garbanzos), and what you prepare from them. Fermented and dried foods are close to fresh foods because they have undergone very little processing. Fermentation actually makes them healthier and more easily digestible, so sauerkraut and miso are naturally enriched with vitamins; our ancestors survived on them in bitter winters when no fresh produce was available. Freezing is an acceptable—but not perfect—modern way of preserving some freshness. Microwaving destroys too many phytonutrients; thaw and reheat in a lidded pot.

Why is fresh, organic food more healthful than processed, microwaved, fortified, enriched, canned, old, rancid, stale, milled food? Whole organic food contains more life-giving phytonutrients than produce that is grown conventionally. Phytonutrients are those special chemicals built up in the plant from water, soil, and sunlight. At one time, researchers thought they were not important for health. Now we are linking the diseases called "civilized" to the absence of phytonutrients in the Standard American Diet ("SAD"): obesity, diabetes, high blood pressure, high cholesterol, heart disease, arthritis, depression, cancer—the list is endless. Phytonutrients are anti-inflammatory, given to us as presents from the plant world—hundreds of them in a single

FOODS HIGH IN PHYTONUTRIENTS

The following foods are very high in phytonutrients. It is not a list of the "top ten best" foods, but it just shows the variety. And we haven't yet explored and researched even the smallest amounts of plant foods available on earth: phytonutrients are in *all* plants.

Apple
Apricot
Aronia
Artichoke
Avocado
Beans
Black currant
Blueberries
Broccoli
Brussels sprouts
Cabbage
Carrots
Cauliflower
Chard, red and
    green
Citrus fruits
Cocoa
Collard greens
Cranberries
Dandelion greens
Eggplant
Elderberries
Garbanzo beans
Garlic
Green tea

Kale
Kohlrabi
Lentils
Mango
Mushrooms
Nuts and seeds
Onion
Papaya
Peas
Peppers, hot and
    sweet
Pink grapefruit
Pomegranate
Pu-erh tea
Pumpkin
Red grapes
Rooibos tea
Rose hips
Sea-buckthorn
Spinach
Squash
Sweet potato
Tomato
Watermelon

plant. In fact, organic food contains about one-third more than conventional, mostly because the soil in conventional agriculture has been deadened and depleted by chemical fertilizers. The health benefits of phytonutrients go beyond vitamins and minerals, and to this day we certainly have not discovered all of them.

The benefits of phytonutrients are transferred to animals that eat them, eventually to our meats and poultry. Organic lamb, for instance, has a very high vitamin C content because lambs are usually thrown out on the pasture soon after birth. They don't get extra feed or antibiotics and hormones. All summer, they feed on untreated meadows. That is why their meat brims with the goods of sun-drenched, natural pastures. Unfortunately, even most of our organic meats are not grass-fed but grain-fed. Grains are unnatural to cows. What we then eat is an animal that was not healthy to begin with. Interestingly, we usually don't eat predators and scavengers (cats, dogs, hyenas, vultures)—they are too far removed from the original, health-giving phytonutrients. And if we eat them—like lobster and shrimp that are the scavengers of the ocean floor—they usually come with a warning not to eat them too frequently. Omnivores, like pigs, fall into the category between grass-eaters and predators, and some cultures shun their meat too.

In addition to phytonutrients, fresh, organic food is more healthful because:

- Fresh, organic food contains lower levels of pesticides, herbicides, and in the case of meats and poultry, lower levels of hormones, antibiotics, and meat fresheners.
- Fresh, organic food contains all the ingredients that correspond to our genetic needs, handed down to us from our evolutionary ancestors.
- Organic, whole foods fuel mitochondria—those cell organs that act as the energy factories in your body. Phytonutrients feed directly into mitochondria, counteracting one of the most common complaints of our times: lack of energy.

- Your body recognizes fresh, organic food as food, whereas it does not recognize many modern adulterated or entirely artificial molecules.
- Fresh, organic food contains good fats, good carbohydrates, and balanced proteins, naturally, taking the "thinking" out of what to eat.
- Fresh, organic food slows down the rate at which the blood sugar levels rise and therefore reduces insulin production. Sugar from the original source—plants—enters your blood slower, since the sugar is only available after plant cell walls have been broken down. Refined sugar and high-fructose corn syrup, in contrast, are available within seconds, swamping your system and acting as a poison—with the long-term consequence of "civilized" diseases.
- Fresh, organic food is naturally full of fiber and therefore lowers cholesterol.
- You must chew fresh, organic food more thoroughly, increasing saliva production and triggering digestive juices adequately. By contrast, junk food can be gobbled down, leaving your stomach and bowel overwhelmed and burdened.
- Fresh, organic food leads to less calorie intake, because chewing and high fiber contents trigger earlier satiety, making you feel full longer. It satisfies your body's needs for phytonutrients in ways that macaroni and cheese cannot.
- Fresh, organic foods increase the bulk of stool, so it passes through the bowel faster, normalizing constipation and diarrhea. They also bind toxins and remove them faster from your gut. You won't need extra bran.
- Fresh, organic foods boost your immune strength, provide some natural antibiotics, and decrease inflammation. In fact, decreasing inflammation is the whole point because lower inflammation will reduce "civilized," degenerative diseases including cancer.

Inflammatory and Anti-Inflammatory Foods

Besides freshness, the second most important quality in foods is their anti-inflammatory activity, which is closely linked to phytonutrients. Look at different foods as the *good guys* and the *bad guys*: *anti-inflammatory* and *inflammatory* foods. Nearly everything whole and fresh is anti-inflammatory. Everything artificial promotes inflammation, especially refined sugars and starches, milk products, and hydrogenated fats (trans fats). Inflammation is a reaction in your cells causing redness, swelling, heat, and pain. It can occur on the skin or inside the body, affecting joints, muscles, and internal organs. A pimple is a perfect example of an inflammation. A bloated abdomen is too. Inflammation, often caused by bad-guy food, is at the root of pain and most chronic diseases, including headaches, diabetes, high blood pressure, arthritis, asthma, hay fever, dementia, and even certain cancers. The good guys heal you by reducing inflammation.

Inflammation is caused by infection, irritation, and/or injury. Often food is the original irritator, either because it is unhealthful to start with or because you personally have developed an allergy and need to avoid that food. (Often, the two are related.)

Many plants are anti-inflammatory—and therefore good for you—because they contain many natural compounds (phytonutrients) that act as anti-inflammatory agents. The more you mix and rotate your fruits and vegetables, the more you benefit from the good guys and the less likely you are to develop a food allergy from overexposure to a single food item.

A Guide to Inflammatory and Anti-Inflammatory Foods

Here is a comparison of foods and preparation methods that are anti-inflammatory (good for you) and inflammatory (could cause problems, especially if you eat too much of them):

Anti-Inflammatory	Inflammatory
Fresh, unprocessed (as grown)	Old, rancid, moldy, processed, microwaved, skimmed, enhanced, canned, adulterated
Fruit	Excessive meats and poultry; dairy
Vegetables (non-nightshade)	Nightshade vegetables (tomato, potato, bell and hot peppers, eggplant)
Herbs	Many drugs and medications (but you may need them)
Water, herbal teas	Soft drinks, milk, juices, etc.
Water	Dehydration
Most plant oils (best is olive oil, especially organic extra-virgin olive oil and organic coconut oil), nut oils (if not rancid), especially those rich in omega-3 fatty acids (nut oils, except coconut oil, should not be heated)	Animal fats, many commercial branded oils, vegetable shortening, corn oil, palm oil
Uncooked and cooked at low heat (steaming, boiling, simmering, braising)	Fried, baked, grilled, and broiled at high temperatures
Soy foods (to a degree)	Dairy products (milk, cheese, yogurt)
Nuts and dried fruit (without added sugar)	Candies, most chocolates, "health" bars
Naturally sweet fruit	Sugars, artificial sweeteners
Whole foods	Artificial molecules

Anti-Inflammatory	Inflammatory
No preservatives	Preservatives like nitrites, benzoic acid
No artificial additives	Artificial additives like dyes, preservatives, flavors, MSG, etc.
Grass-fed meats	Corn-fed meats
Nuts (if you are not allergic)	Peanuts (they are legumes, not nuts; should be eaten sparingly)
Fish, especially seawater	Excessive meats and poultry
Nonhydrogenated fats	Hydrogenated or partially hydrogenated fats (trans fats)
Food your body likes	Food your body reacts adversely to

Some foods are neither inflammatory nor anti-inflammatory. Grains, for instance, including rice, fall into this neutral category for most people. But some people react to grains (especially gluten-containing grains), and then the grains act like inflammatory agents and are toxic, because wheat, soy, and other grains contain inflammatory substances called lectins. Lectins play some beneficial roles in the body, but mostly they cause inflammation. All seeds, including wheat, legumes, and nuts, are high in lectins and should be avoided if you react to them.

Vegetables from the nightshade family (tomato, potato, bell and hot peppers, eggplant) all contain another inflammatory substance called solanine. They are harder for some people to tolerate than for others. We're all slightly different genetically, with different metabolisms, so we have different food requirements that cannot be neatly prescribed by a doctor. You have to listen to your own body and discover what is best for you. You can figure out your personal "food reaction profile" by observing yourself closely after you eat and keeping a journal of your reactions to foods. Listen when your body speaks to you! (Chapter 16 gives hints about which ways your body speaks to you if it doesn't like the food you are eating.)

CHAPTER 15

THE JOY OF EATING
MAKING LIFE-AFFIRMING CHOICES

Now that you have heard about the importance of fresh food, this chapter will give you some tips about how to eat and how to eat well and make the right food choices for *your* body.

Nourish Yourself with Joy

The following guidelines will help you get the most out of your meals:

- **Celebrate meals instead of foods.** Try to avoid eating alone; instead, share your meals with friends and family. Always set the table simply but beautifully. Add a flower or a candle. Use your best china every day—who are you saving it for?
- **Eat regularly; don't skip meals.** Have at least three meals per day, five are even better. Children as well as the elderly and people of light constitutions might need more frequent meals. Never skip breakfast, as it starts your day on a wrong note. The timing of your food intake is important, because it has to be in harmony with your daily hormonal cycle. Breakfast should come after your morning routine of grooming and mental preparation for the day. Dinner should not be so late that your stomach is still full when you go to

bed (at least three hours before bedtime); best before sunset. Nighttime snacks are out of the question, because your body needs the nightly fast to repair the damage done the previous day, to cleanse itself, and to recover strength for the next day.

- **Eat in leisure, quiet, and joy and attentively.** Don't quarrel or fight at the table. Reading, listening to the radio, or watching television distracts you from appreciating the beauty, aromas, and taste of the victuals and the care the cook has put into preparing this meal—and leads to poor digestion. Try exploring the different textures with your tongue and gums, feeling the crispness between your teeth, letting the softness run down your throat. Taste sweet and sour, salty and bitter, and savor the differences, harmonies, and unexpected disharmonies.

- **Chew slowly.** Put down your fork between bites. (But there's no need to make chewing an ideology.)

- **Posture when eating is important.** Slumping squeezes your stomach. Lying down leads to heartburn and reflux.

- **Consider saying grace when you sit down for a meal.** The key is gratitude. Water and the soil, animals and plants are feeding you in an eternal cycle of life. Feel connected to the whole earth.

- **Eat to nourish yourself.** Remember the saying "location, location, location" when you want to buy a house? My mantra for food is "vegetables, vegetables, vegetables." The bulk of your food should be vegetables (and fruit, whole grains, legumes and nuts—plant fare). At least half of the vegetables should be cooked. Wash fruits and vegetables thoroughly and rinse well. Raw food is harder to digest, especially for people of slight constitution. Experiment with how much plant food your body needs. Different body types have different tolerances for meats, fats, and raw plant foods. Intolerances of quantities and qualities might show in dyspepsia, heartburn, abdominal pain and discomfort, bloating, belching, and increased gas.

- **Eat in moderation.** Sebastian Kneipp said: big dinners fill coffins. Paavo Airola, a European naturopath, put it this way: practice *systematic undereating*. That's not the same as starving; it means to stop when your needs have been met, long before you are stuffed. Your digestive tract has an optimal capacity; beyond that, digestion is sluggish and ineffective. At the other extreme, if you starve yourself, your body shifts to starvation mode and will hold on desperately to every calorie, making weight loss more difficult. Observe when and why you eat, and if you detect an unhealthy pattern, look for remedies (see Chapter 16).

- **Remember that food is only one of the Five Water Essentials.** In this section, we focus on food, but food is not all. It is far better to enjoy an occasional unhealthful meal and the hospitality of friends than to sit in front of your correct muesli or salad and be unhappy. It is important, however, that your refrigerator and your pantry at home contain *only* healthful food.

- **Vegetarian or not?** Vegetarian fare might not be for everybody because each person's heritage is different. Experiment and observe for yourself. Build your meals around vegetables, not around meat, poultry, or fish—they should be like an afterthought. For my patients, I usually recommend fish three times a week, vegetarian three times a week, and meat once a week.

- **Remember that falling off the wagon is normal.** Do not get upset when you break your rules, but do so with joy and abandon. Celebrate the few occasions when you indulge (definitely not more than once a month!). Use the opportunity to observe what it does to your body—write it down! And then resume the healthy life.

GOOD NEWS ABOUT CHOCOLATE

Cocoa leads the list of foods brimming with phytonutrients. Notice, I didn't say a chocolate bar. But chocolate is more healthful than you might think. It tops the list of foods high in phytonutrients—way ahead of broccoli. Among other benefits, it works against depression, probably via a mitochondrial boost. It gives you a gentle lift-me-up like a caffeinated beverage. Yes, chocolate contains fats and calories, so use it sparingly—but savor each little piece!

Chocolate's unhealthful qualities come from additives: sugar and high-fructose corn syrup, milk and milk products, and cheap flavorings. But an organic dark chocolate (containing at least 70 percent cacao) that is dairy-free and sweetened lightly with cane or beet sugar is well worth the extra expense. Or buy baker's chocolate. It's quite bitter but has no nutritional spoilers and is cheap. Use unsweetened cocoa for hot chocolate, and make it with soy milk and water. And in the future, look out for new products that will offer chocolate without added ingredients.

Drink Water, of Course!

As you know, water is essential for the health and well-being of every person. Here are some of the many benefits of drinking fresh, clean water:

- Water quenches thirst. The awareness of thirst diminishes with age, so older people need to be mindful of drinking enough every day.
- It brings moisture and nutrients to your organs.

- It has antiaging qualities.
- It flushes out impurities, detoxifying your body.
- It beautifies your skin and smoothes out wrinkles.
- It improves brain function.
- It lubricates joints.
- It regulates body temperature.
- It increases energy.
- It releases stress, because dehydration is one of the biggest stressors for the body. Nothing functions well without water's soothing, renewing qualities.
- It helps reduce weight gain when drunk half an hour before a meal by leading to an earlier feeling of fullness.
- It prevents kidney stones.
- Natural spring water contains essential minerals: bicarbonates (which regulate acidity), calcium (strengthens bones), chloride (regulates acidity), fluoride (protects your teeth from cavities), iron (prevents anemia), magnesium (essential for your heart, bones, and temperature regulation), potassium (important for heart and muscles), sodium (balances water distribution), and zinc (helps bones, immunity, wound healing, and diabetes control). These minerals can be picked up by the water as it travels through different soils and sediments. Therefore, water from different springs might have very different mineral contents. Nothing is as good as a pure spring or a deep (tested) well.

Water Consumption Tips

Use these water consumption tips to get the most out of the water you're drinking:

- **Don't overdo it.** You need seven cups of water as a baseline—more in hot weather and with exercise. There is no need to walk around with a bottle in your hand all day. If you drink too much, you deplete your body of electrolytes (salts)

and tax your heart and kidneys. You are getting enough
liquid if your urine is light-colored and plentiful.

- **Bottled is not always best.** Often, you are not sure of
the source, and the bottling process and the bottles use up
precious resources. A better alternative is a simple water
filter—either on the counter or under it, attached to your
faucet.

- **Fresh foods contain water, too.** Eat plenty of fruit and
vegetables. Not only do they contain 80 to 95 percent
water, but the water is in the purest form because the plants
have filtered out impurities. While herbal teas, soups, and
carbonated waters are also good, nothing surpasses fresh,
clean water. Beverages, including teas, even herbal teas, are
not the same as plain water: they also need to be processed
by the liver. If at first you do not like the taste of plain water;
learn to like it by preparing your herbal teas thinner and
thinner, or by diluting fruit juices more and more. Coffee
and alcohol are diuretics, so they count for about half of
their fluid only.

- **Think about juices as you think about refined sugar or
white flour.** Juices deliver too much of a good thing in too
short a time for our bodies to be able to deal with it. For
millions of years, we adapted to eating a whole ripe seasonal
fruit and chewing it well, and then drinking spring water.
We are not made for the onslaught of orange juice, daily. If,
occasionally, you want to indulge yourself with *fresh* juice,
dilute it at least by half with good, pure water. Exceptions are
herbal juices.

What About Dairy?

When I was a child, my father, who was also a doctor, told me a
story about a famous world traveler who arrived in a Far Eastern
village after an exhausted ride over the mountains and, through

his interpreter, asked for a glass of milk. It took hours before the beverage arrived. But then it surprised the traveler by its unusually delicious taste. "Which animal gives such sweet milk?" the traveler inquired. After a lot of concerned silence and bashful avoidance, the answer came: "A woman."

Milk in ancient Asia was not perceived as a food for people—except for infants. That is why the traveler's request sent the village into confusion. In the last few years, I have seen our local Chinese supermarket go from offering no cow's milk to stocking the usual suspects—skim milk, yogurt, cottage cheese—while the area for fresh soy milk is getting smaller, thereby setting up the mostly Chinese customers for all of our Western diseases like diabetes, heart disease, acne, indigestion, arthritis, and so on.

Milk and dairy products are generally not appropriate for us to consume. During a certain period in our history, cow's milk was a godsend for babies and children who otherwise would have died of starvation. But now, in an affluent Western country, there is no need to have dairy on your menu—as much as the dairy industry wants you to believe otherwise.

Research has linked milk to all kinds of diseases, either as the cause or an aggravating factor. Hay fever, asthma, bronchitis, chronic sinusitis, ear infections, eczema, food allergies, diabetes—the list goes on and on. Many people have a lactose deficiency, which makes it impossible to digest lactose, the milk sugar, resulting in gastrointestinal disturbances. Don't try to counter it with the use of lactose-free milk; just skip dairy altogether.

What About the Calcium Connection?

Dairy products are promoted as a needed calcium source only because our usual Western diet is too high in protein. If you digest proteins, the end product is an acidic metabolic product that needs calcium as a buffer in our systems. Your body takes the calcium from your bones because there is plenty of it. But over a lifetime, you deplete even that abundant source of calcium, and the result is osteoporosis (thinning of the bones). Fractured hips and other broken bones in the elderly are a huge national disaster. If we would moderate our intake of protein from animal sources, particularly meats and dairy products, we would more likely do just fine with the available calcium in vegetables—for instance, in greens, beans, nuts, and whole grains. Besides, bones need many more minerals than calcium—like boron, selenium, magnesium, manganese, and so forth.

What About Soy Milk?

Sadly, soy is not a perfect food either. Yes, it has good phyto-estrogens (but so have most beans, lentils, and garbanzos), but it inhibits the thyroid. For that reason, try to combine soy with seaweed. Also, in most forms—soy milk, tofu, health food snacks—soy is highly processed and therefore not recommended. Furthermore, the soybean crop is often genetically manipulated and overfertilized. Occasionally, soy is OK, but it is really not a health food.

What About Vitamins and Other Supplements?

With the best of foods, you wouldn't need to supplement with anything; it would be all in the fresh, water-bursting plants, grown on good soil. Since we are not living in the best of all worlds, here are some tips:

- There are some diseases for which you urgently need a vitamin pill or shot (pernicious anemia with vitamin B_{12} deficiency, for instance). If your physician prescribes a vitamin to you, don't stop taking it unless you have discussed it. But insist that she check your lab numbers from time to time.

- What applies to juices applies also to supplements: too much of a good thing taken in too short a time might wreak more havoc than good. Several studies have shown that food filled with vitamins is healthful (fights cancer, for instance), whereas vitamin supplements are not.
- People have tons of unfinished vitamin bottles at home— you might too. There probably is body wisdom at work: you don't need all that stuff. I have taken many more people off vitamins than I have started. If you feel sorry to throw out unused, expensive supplements, take one from time to time. Your body's thinking of a vitamin or mineral pill might mean that you need one.
- Don't ever think a supplement can replace fresh food. It can't.

Sebastian Kneipp said the path to health leads through the kitchen—not through the pharmacy. I concede that, of the Five Water Essentials, good nutrition is the hardest to maintain, because cooking from scratch cannot be done in two minutes. But, even as a busy doctor, I always cooked for my family, because I knew I could not give my family more love than in healthy meals.

To keep it simple, I will share a single recipe that can be used for stir-fry, soup, or stew and is different every time you put it on the table.

This stir-fry recipe can be changed into a soup just by filling up with water—or into a stew by throwing the ingredients in a slow-cooking pot and cooking on low for several hours.

Serve with brown rice, quinoa, millet, buckwheat, amaranth, lentils, beans, garbanzos, chana dal, or split peas.

Always serve with a salad. Dressing: olive oil, lemon or vinegar, black pepper, salt, and ground herbs like thyme, oregano, savory, or rosemary.

DR. ALEXA'S STIR-FRY

1. Sauté some onions and garlic in olive or coconut oil in a large pan.
2. Choose seven vegetables. Wash organic fare; peel all conventional produce, if possible. Add the vegetables in the order of their cooking time (longest cooking time goes in first). For instance, parsnips, celery root, celery stalk, mushrooms, carrots, zucchini, then snap peas. Keep a lid on. Use a different combination every time. In the market, I go for what is organic, fresh, and cheap.
3. Add herbs and spices freely—fresh or dried. Add black pepper and salt to taste (I use herbal salt, and very little).
4. You may add fish, shrimp, ground beef, pork, or lamb to the dish. Or you can broil it in the oven. Keep portions small.
5. Serve soon; don't overcook.

CHAPTER 16

WEIGHT LOSS
NEVER DIET AGAIN

W hen it came to weight, Sebastian Kneipp believed in one primary law of nature: the food that goes into the body creates the body. If you feed your body with pizza, ice cream, and doughnuts, you will get a pizza-ice-cream-and-doughnut body. If you feed it a bit better, your body will get (and be and feel and look) a bit better. If you feed it a lot better, you will reap health and well-being in every one of the gazillions of cells in your body.

If you ever have—and who has not?—tried to lose weight on a crash diet, only to gain it back in no time—and more to boot!—here is a plan that will never leave you hungry and that needs no calorie counting. There is only one rule you need to follow: everything that goes into your mouth should be fresh and healthful. Always be mindful of the other four Water Essentials: cold water, movement, herbs, and the natural order and flow of life.

Over and over, I have seen the health-by-water weight loss program work with my patients to fight weight gain and obesity. I have also seen it prevent and even cure the deadly syndrome X—the triad of diabetes, high blood pressure, and elevated blood fats, along with their loyal companions, arthritis, fatigue, and depression.

Keep in mind that no diet is right for everybody. No book can tell you the right foods for your particular body. But this book can help you figure it out for yourself. Forget about the newest fad diet, and learn what is good for *you*. I can give you some hints and some basic facts, but the proof is in the pudding: if a food doesn't agree with you, don't eat it! For example, if a food gives you heartburn, don't eat it. Doctors easily prescribe medications for heartburn. But covering up the symptom does not change the fact that the food you ate does not agree with your system. It is neither normal nor healthy to have heartburn. Not only does disagreeable food damage your stomach and your esophagus, it also might produce inflammation at other places in your body, with long-term consequences. The same goes for every other food-related symptom: headaches, joint pains, bloating, and so forth.

Diet and Nutrition

What is the difference between diet and nutrition? *Nutrition* is about everything that goes into your mouth, all day, every day. *Diets* are short-term variations of food intake patterns, most for the purpose of reducing weight, some for certain diseases. Short-term diets, especially for weight loss, do not have long-term effects—as studies have shown, and many people have found out to their dismay. But if you use the water-based Freshness Pyramid as your guide (see Chapter 14), you will have a much easier time losing weight than if you try to stick to a "diet."

If you feel unhappy with your present nutritional state—and chances are you do, because more than 50 percent of Americans are overweight—try to slowly change what you eat by using the freshness guide to healthful food. Obviously, this includes beverages, too. Learning about food will be an ongoing process—like everything else in life—and this chapter will give you some guidelines for losing weight permanently, without "dieting."

FOOD ALLERGIES AND WEIGHT GAIN

Because they trigger inflammation in your body, food allergies may cause excess weight gain, mostly from swelling. If you find yourself excessively thirsty during or after a meal, your weight gain may be caused by a food allergy. (Other causes may include diseases, particularly diabetes, so consult with your doctor.) Allergies and food intolerances make you crave and binge, too. The most common culprits are usually foods we eat too often: sugar, corn, high-fructose corn syrup and other corn-derived products (most modern food additives!), wheat and other gluten grains (barley, rye, oats), beef (probably because it is corn-fed), citrus, nuts and seeds, soy, peanuts, shellfish, eggs, chocolate (most often the additives cause problems, not cocoa itself), and fish.

Therefore, a first step in permanent weight loss is to try to determine which foods you may be allergic or intolerant to. Allergies are difficult to diagnose and to confirm. Even if you or your doctor suspects an allergy, many physicians are not educated to recognize food allergies and food intolerances. If self-observation does not solve the problem, seek help from a trained allergist, since many of the signs and symptoms of food allergies can also stem from a myriad of diseases. In addition to excessive thirst, here are some other clues to possible food allergies:

- **General:** fatigue, feeling faint, lassitude, general weakness, food cravings, binges, sudden hunger pangs, jitters, hypoglycemia, alcoholism, obesity, weight loss, extreme weight fluctuations
- **Skin:** itchiness, rashes, red spots, dandruff, hives
- **Mind:** sleepiness, confusion, anxiety, depression, lethargy, hyperactivity, aggression, difficulties focusing, mood swings, irritability, emotional turmoil, sleeplessness

- **Head and neck:** burning or tickling sensations in mouth or throat, headaches, sinus problems, dizziness, difficulty hearing, ringing in the ear, itchy or watery eyes, bleeding gums, canker sores, chronic eye infections, chronic ear infections, recurrent sore throat, hoarseness
- **Chest:** asthma, lung congestion, chronic cough, difficulty breathing, palpitations, rapid heartbeat
- **Abdomen:** bloating, dyspepsia, heartburn, stomach pains, diarrhea or constipation, cramps, gas, nausea, vomiting, prolonged fullness
- **Arms and legs:** heaviness in limbs, bursitis, tendonitis, joint pains, arthritis, phlebitis, weakness, swelling of hands, feet, or ankles
- **Pelvis:** urinary problems, burning on urination, genital itch, anal itch

Any of these symptoms and signs can also be caused by serious medical illness. Food allergies should only be considered when serious disease has been ruled out by your physician.

Whether you are trying to lose weight or not, do not ignore your reactions to food. Listen to what your body is trying to tell you! A pain or a discomfort is the only language your body has to communicate with you. Shutting it up with pain pills will do nothing to cure the root cause. If you don't listen now, symptoms will only get worse.

Weight Loss Tip 1:
Cleanse Your Body with a Water-Based Fast

Most cultures have a time of fasting in the rhythm of the year. For Christians it is Lent (the time before Easter); for Muslims,

Ramadan; and for Jews, several days during the year, especially at Yom Kippur. In religious practices, fasting is a spiritual discipline. But religion aside, regular fasting is also a great device for detoxification, a first step to losing weight permanently. Once your body loses these toxins, you will find it a lot easier to lose weight.

Traditionally, we had a little fast automatically built into every day: between supper (which used to be a light meal) and breakfast, we would not eat. Nothing. The very word *breakfast* is "break fast." I find it interesting that in medieval times in Europe, people often had only two meals. During the nightly fast, the body repairs and cleanses itself. Damaged muscles, stretched tissues, accumulated toxins, broken DNA, sluggish immune system—they all need daily repair.

But our modern lifestyles—late dining, TV munching, and raiding the fridge after midnight—wreak havoc on our innate biological rhythms. We have lost our repair and cleansing time. Weight gain is not the only result. A worn-out immune system that cannot fight infections and cancers is the price we pay for our mindless indulgences.

Besides keeping the nightly fast, committing to fasting regularly will increase your well-being. I advise all of my healthy patients to fast about one day a month, according to the guidelines that follow. But if ailments like diabetes, arthritis, or allergies have already crept up on you, I recommend fasting for one day each week until they feel better. Fasting is especially valuable for people who are overweight and/or have heavy muscle mass. Thin or weak people should be careful about fasting.

CAUTION: If you struggle with anorexia or any other wasting disease, fasting is not for you. As with all suggestions in this book, check with your doctor before embarking on a fast.

The Benefits of Fasting

Did you know that carnivores such as cats and dogs usually fast several days between meals in the wild? Obviously, they do this when they don't find prey, but in addition, their systems seem to get overloaded with protein (which is harder to digest than fat and carbohydrates), so they need a rest period. Herbivores like cows and sheep are always eating. They do not do well when deprived of food, as any farmer will tell you. We humans, as omnivores, are in the middle. Vegetarians need it less urgently than meat eaters, but fasting from time to time does most of us good.

Fasting offers a variety of benefits:

- Weight loss (mainly water)
- Detoxifying
- Renewal and repair of your cells and muscles
- Mental clarity
- Greater body awareness, as you become more attuned to when your body is and is not truly hungry
- Gratitude for simpler, fresher food

Preparing for a One-Day Fast

Anything longer than a one-day fast should be done under supervision of a physician. Do not expect to lose weight during the fasting day. You mainly lose water and toxins. But because you have been deprived of food and taken out of mindless munching habits, your appetite will be smaller, and you will be more aware of what goes into your body and how you feel after eating. And that should lead to weight loss.

The fast I am proposing is a vegetable broth fast. I find it superior to a juice fast because vegetables are alkaline and don't bother an empty stomach as acidic fruits do. The broth—which is made with water, of course—will soothe your stomach. You can alternate broth with fresh filtered water and herbal teas.

Start by preparing broth in a huge pot. (Avoid aluminum. Aluminum has been linked to such diseases as Alzheimer's, osteoporosis, gastrointestinal problems, interference with the metabolism of calcium, extreme nervousness, anemia, headaches, decreased liver and kidney function, memory loss, speech problems, softening of the bones, and aching muscles.) Throw into it everything vegetable that lingers in your fridge, with the exception of nightshades (tomato, potato, bell and hot peppers, eggplant). Add herbs, fresh or dried. Onions and garlic give your soup a delicious sweetness. Don't add salt, spices, or any meat or fish or eggs. Add enough water to barely cover the vegetables. Cook for at least an hour; it makes a delicious broth. During your fast, do not eat the vegetables; just drink the flavorful water. (If you want, you can eat the vegetables after the fast as discussed later.)

Your last meal before the fast should be light, preferably vegetarian. You can start anytime; most people prefer to begin in the morning. I have found it helpful to start after a transatlantic flight, when my system is out of order anyway, and I crave a cleansing after German liverwurst and airline fare. While I unpack my suitcase and get reacquainted with my cat and family, water the flowers, and put in the first load of laundry, I drink herbal teas. I prepare my broth and go to bed very early. When I wake up the next morning, I have already completed about eighteen hours of fasting—a big motivator to pull through the entire twenty-four hours.

During the Fast

Fasting might make you feel worse before you feel better, because it brings toxins and waste products into your circulation. You might experience headaches, severe chilliness, bad breath, nausea, and lethargy, especially during longer fasts.

Follow these guidelines while you're fasting:

- Drink only water, herbal teas, and vegetable broth. *Do not drink:* coffee, black or green tea, milk, soft drinks or juices.
- Your first herbal tea at the beginning of your fast should be a laxative (such as ginger, fenugreek, or sweet violets). Magnesium salts also work for emptying your bowels. Do not use too much—a single good bowel movement is sufficient.
- Drink broth whenever you are hungry. You can add water and boil your vegetables again as the day goes on; your broth will still be palatable with the third or fifth steeping. Drink in small sips; chew the broth to stimulate saliva production.
- Light exercise such as walking, swimming, bicycling, yoga, or tai chi will help you through the day when you feel cold, tired, sluggish, and/or depressed.
- Keep warm, rest when you need to, and focus on the positive outcome of your fast.
- Experienced fasters can work while fasting, but I would not recommend it for a beginner. Take this time to listen to your body and your soul.
- Recruit a friend who will fast with you. Sharing the experience makes it easier.
- Do not smoke during your fast. In fact, a fast is a wonderful way to quit smoking.

If fasting seems daunting, start by replacing a single meal with vegetable broth. That alone will have a good effect on digestion and cravings. I prefer to substitute a dinner. With the normal night fast, that already gives you a good twelve hours of fasting—time for your body to repair.

Break the fast with a light meal of fruit and/or a salad. Or you can eat the vegetables from the broth. I usually replace the water several times; so the vegetables are devoid of nutritional value. But they still give you bulk and fiber. To the last bowl of overcooked vegetables, I add some olive oil. This is a good way to restart regular food. You may also just discard the vegetables; truth be told, they are quite tasteless.

CAUTION: If you have the following conditions, fasting is not advisable:

- Anorexia
- Depression
- Being underweight (BMI below ideal)
- Acute viral illness
- Fever
- Wasting diseases (tuberculosis, AIDS, late-stage cancer)
- Anxiety

Weight Loss Tip 2:
Cleanse Your Body Gently Using Herbs

If fasting does not agree with you, there is always gentle cleansing with herbs. For a month, use the following herbs (after checking with your doctor):

- Milk thistle
- Dandelion
- Stinging nettle

Stinging nettle and dandelion are mild diuretics, helping to detox your body via the kidneys. Milk thistle does the same through the liver and the bowels. I prefer the liquid herbs in a tincture, rather than capsules. Use one dropperful of each herb, three times a day, diluted in a cup of warm water.

After a month, give your body a rest of at least a month before you start the cycle again. Don't use this treatment more than two months without consulting your physician or a knowledgeable herbalist.

Also, try to incorporate cilantro into your food (in soups, salads, stews, and so on). It contains many vital phytonutrients and may even help lower cholesterol. And take chlorella (either alone or in a probiotic). Chlorella brings out toxic substances from your tissues into your blood, and cilantro binds them so that they can be eliminated.

Weight Loss Tip 3: Drink Water Before Meals

Drinking a glass of water half an hour before each meal will help you lose weight by filling you up and also will take away waste, toxic matter, and excess salts from your body. We die of thirst much faster than of starvation, and we lose about two cups of water per day alone by breathing. Water sustains your body without adding fat or sugar or calories. Begin with seven cups of water a day as a baseline—more in hot weather and if you exercise. Drink it from a beautiful cup.

Weight Loss Tip 4: Go Shopping After You've Eaten

Do not go food shopping when you are hungry. Even though it is good to stick to a shopping list, I never go into the store with a completely preconceived notion of what I will be cooking—I look for what's fresh and what's cheap. However, if I try this approach when I am hungry, I buy unhealthful foods, just because I hear my stomach rumbling. Eat before venturing down those super-market aisles.

Weight Loss Tip 5: Buy Fresh, Organic Foods

What I choose is based on what looks freshest. I take the freshest fish, the freshest vegetables, bursting with water. And if I have the choice, I buy organic: good food builds a better body.

Weight Loss Tip 6:
Avoid Refined Sugar, White Starches, and Juices

Avoid refined sugar, white starches (simple carbohydrates), and undiluted and sweetened juices altogether. Our digestive system is not able to handle them in this unnatural state. (Even if they were originally derived from natural sources, they are now processed, altered foods.) Refined sugar enters the bloodstream too fast and overpowers the insulin-producing cells in the pancreas. White flour contains only the inner starchy core of the wheat grain after the outer hulls have been removed. White flour is totally devoid of vitamins and minerals. Essentially, starches are nothing else than long sugar chains, easily clipped by digestive juices and ready to overwhelm and poison your body. Sugar and white flour are simple carbohydrates, which our system does not handle well, especially if you are trying to lose weight.

Undiluted juices, much like refined sugar, are also unnatural for our bodies and bring too much good stuff in too short a time into your system. I have thought about this point a lot: how unhealthful are juices? I do not want you to buy a juicer and drink fruit juices, because it is unnatural to our digestive system. But all too many people are barely taking in any vegetables and fruit. What if the juicer captures their fancy and starts them on a healthier lifestyle? Who am I to tell them not to start their day with a vegetable or fruit drink? If you are like most Americans, you are eating a very unhealthful diet as it is, and making your own juices might be a big step toward healthier nutrition. But eat the pulp, too! If you are already eating quite sensibly, then a juicer will not be what you want. It is better to chew your fruit and vegetables.

Common Reasons Why People Are Overweight

The first step to losing weight is finding out why you eat too much of the wrong foods. Here are some possible reasons to consider:

- **Government diet recommendations:** These recommendations have been proven to lead to weight gain. Government recommendations include foods that are low in fat and high in simple carbohydrates, and they include dairy products, which as we've seen, lead to weight gain and not weight loss. Good fats nourish you and prevent early hunger. I noticed that I need more fat than most people, and I do eat more, but only *good* fats.
- **Stress:** Being overly anxious or stressed out contributes to weight gain because, when you're stressed, your body produces a substance called cortisol, which leads to uncontrollable hunger and overeating.
- **Boredom:** Not leading an active, engaging life may lead to weight gain if you eat as a way of occupying yourself when you feel that you have nothing else to do.
- **Loneliness, sadness, and depression:** These are frequent causes of weight gain. Many people try to alleviate the sadness in their lives with food—and then bad food increases sadness and depression. Furthermore, some of the medications that treat depression and anxiety contribute to weight gain as a side effect.
- **The media:** TV and movies tout an ideal of impossible slimness (bordering on anorexia, from a doctor's eye) and barrage you with ads for unhealthful food at the same time, creating unhealthy body shame. Slogans like "You deserve it!" deceive you; you don't deserve obesity and ill health.
- **Poor eating habits:** Skipping meals (especially breakfast!) leads to overeating later in the day and midnight foraging at the refrigerator.
- **Weight loss diets:** Physicians now mostly agree that diet-induced weight loss is only transient. You nearly always regain more than you weighed before. The deprivation of a weight loss diet leads to ravenous hunger and/or cravings for depleted nutrients.

- **Weight:** Weight gain itself is one reason for weight gain:
  The more you eat, the hungrier you get, due to certain
  chemicals in our brains. That mechanism made it possible
  for cave dwellers to eat the mammoth while it was available
  and store some extra pounds for leaner times. Nowadays, the
  stores, your fridge and pantry are full of "mammoths," and
  the leaner times never arrive.
- **Food addiction:** We are addicted to food, particularly what
  we call "comfort food." Childhood memories and early
  habits make us long for comfort foods, but these foods
  consist mostly of grains, fats, and dairy, all of which contain
  substances that will be turned to morphine-like "feel-good"
  substances in your body.
- **Wrong foods:** These feed the wrong bacteria in your
  bowels, making you crave and binge on foods that feed the
  bad bacteria—a vicious cycle.

If you are trying to lose weight, try to stick to four to five small
meals a day instead of three larger meals, and do not eat every
time food is in sight. If that is too hard, add two snacks of fruit
and raw vegetables.

If you are overweight, you are taking in more calories than
you use up—but the answer does not lie in counting calories. The
answer lies mainly in the kind of food you eat and how often you
eat it. Nobody could gain weight on fruit and vegetables alone. So,
fit in as many fruits and vegetables in your diet as you can. But also
have small amounts of fat and protein in every meal to prevent hunger. In addition, for weight loss, use as many fresh or dried kitchen
herbs (parsley, dill, cilantro, basil, mints, oregano, savory, tarragon,
marjoram, etc.) as you can find. They will provide vitamins and
minerals and come closest to what our forebearers, the cave dwellers, ate. (Learn more about herbs in Part 4 of this book.)

Before you embark on your health-by-water weight loss adven-
ture, ask your physician to check your good and bad cholesterol,

blood sugars (diabetes test), homocysteine and C-reactive protein (markers for heart desease), and thyroid function. And have your vitamin B$_{12}$ checked also. **It is never safe to embark on a weight loss program without your doctor's consent.**

Using All of the Five Water Essentials in Your Weight Loss Program

Weight loss needs to be based on all the Five Water Essentials— not only on food. In addition to everything mentioned already, the following points are important:

- Do not lose more than one to two pounds per month. If you lose weight faster than that, your body goes into starvation mode and will grab on to every single calorie.
- Never ever go hungry—always have a healthful snack, such as seaweed, nuts, avocado, fruit (fresh or dried), or vegetables with you.
- Absolutely do not eat between dinner and breakfast. Your body needs repair time.
- Fill up on vegetables, vegetables, vegetables. Everything else is a side dish.
- All animal fats are unhealthful (except fish), so eat less meat and poultry. Aim for meat (lamb, turkey, chicken, ostrich, beef, beefalo, rabbit, or pork) about once a week, fish (preferably small fish) three times a week, and vegetarian meals three times a week.
- The most unhealthful fats are (partially) hydrogenated fats (trans-fatty acids). They are manufactured for longer shelf life or are formed when food is fried. Absolutely do not eat these.
- Dairy is unnecessary and dangerous. For the transition, try soy or rice milk, *unsweetened*.

- The exact amount and relation of fats, proteins, and complex carbohydrates is different for every person. Therefore, no single diet works for everybody. *Listen to your body*, and find out what gives you enough energy for your day.
- While you still want to lose weight, don't have grains and legumes at dinner, but have plenty of them along with good fat and protein for breakfast and lunch.
- Don't take your diet so seriously that you don't join in when there is a feast and a big party. But don't party every week, and try to be reasonable.
- Hunger versus cravings—know the signs. Food cravings are a sign of food addiction and food allergies. See a knowledgeable doctor.
- Use the scale every morning—but don't obsess about it. Make sure that you are not gaining; that is more important than losing fast. Know that shedding even between two and five pounds changes your metabolic state and improves your health.
- When you need a reward, use fruit and the occasional very small piece of dark chocolate.
- Go on a one-day fast every week until your weight is ideal. Then change to once a month. Although this is more for detoxification than for weight loss, it is important because weight loss flushes toxins from the fat cells into the bloodstream.
- If you fall off the wagon, just get back on without criticizing yourself. No one can eat perfectly all the time.
- Whatever you eat, pay attention and eat it mindfully—don't gobble things down in front of the TV.
- Start exercising. You can do two minutes a day, every day!

PART 4

HERBS

VITAL GREENS, LIQUID MEDICINE

THINK OF HERBS AS EXTRA-STRENGTH PACKAGES OF VEG-etables. They are loaded with vitamins, antioxidants, essential oils, soluble fiber, minerals (including calcium), enzymes, chlorophyll, silica, bitter substances, and innumerable other compounds to boost your health—all the phytonutrients we have talked about before. Water has pulled soil strength into the herbs, and the sun has concentrated these micronutrients more than in vegetables and fruit. Therefore, we use herbs not by the armful, but use them knowledgeably in healing and sprinkle them in or on most of our food, freely and generously. With their fortified sun-and-soil strength, herbs nurture the cells of our bodies.

In medical terms herbs include everything from the plant kingdom that is used for healing purposes: leaves, roots and resins, flowers, stamens, stems, fruit, bark, seeds, berries from trees and shrubs, bulbs, even mushrooms—anything from the vegetation realm. Herbs are the toughies of the plant kingdom, concentrated little medicine bags, developed to ward off parasites and animals. We have evolved for millions of years alongside the herbs of our planet, and our bodies just know how to make use of them. Herbs are nature's keys into the locks of our physiology.

We can harvest nature's green power in teas, for cooking, and in medicinal herbs for good health. Drinking herbal teas and infusions helps meet your daily water quota while giving you vital nutrients and disease-fighting substances at the same time.

Green Means Water: The Source of Life

What makes *green* so beautiful? Why is it that everybody sighs at the sight of a lush green landscape, a garden in bloom—even a painted picture of a natural scene? One could call this an acquired taste, acquired over the millions of years of our evolution. Green, above all, means water, the source of all life. And where there is water, there is food: herbal plants, trees, and bushes with delicious fruits, grains, and—somewhere hidden in the ground but given away by succulent greens on top—savory roots. Green means nourishment also for animals, which in turn may provide food for humans. Green also provides shade from the blistering sun and means there is enough warmth for humankind to thrive; human life is impossible in eternal ice and snow for very long (even the Inuit enjoy a very short summer with some vegetation growth).

Green is not just any color; green is the color of life, the color of the chlorophyll in leaves. Water pulls the benefit of the soil into the herb, but the power of the sun transforms the dead minerals into the stuff of life. Without boring you too much with plant physiology, let me just say that green chlorophyll is the pigment substance that turns light into sugar and starch. Without green plants, we could not exist.

Green plants are not only food for humans and animals. They also replenish oxygen in the air, lower dust and airborne pollutants, and reduce stress by giving us the green environment our ancient physiology obviously craves. Awareness about our innate needs for green has heightened during the last twenty-five years. It has led to "green" trends that include a boom in houseplants (good for your soul and for fresh air), gardening, organic food, and the environmental movement.

The Healing Tradition of Herbs

Herbs have been with humankind forever. The Old Testament exudes heavy whiffs of spices and herbs. During medieval times, Europeans traded for plants from the Mediterranean and the Orient, together with spices, silk, and jewelry. Shamans (traditional healers) all over the world cure with herbs. They did it in prehistoric times, and they still do it now, in indigenous cultures. Likewise, physicians from Hippocrates (circa 460 to circa 377 B.C.) until early in the twentieth century were always herbalists. My father, who became a doctor around 1930, learned botany (and zoology) in medical school, but in the seventies, when I followed in his footsteps, any plant knowledge had been dropped from the curriculum—except for the exciting tidbits that digitalis is derived from foxglove and quinine from the cinchona tree.

During my father's practice, botanical medicine lost its appeal as modern medicine advanced fast, throwing unbelievably effective medications on the market. With the advent of ether and antiseptics in the middle of the nineteenth century, surgery had been improved from sheer butchery to an art and a science. Antibiotics started their victorious years in the 1940s. The Flexner Report—a study of American and Canadian medical education published in 1910 and written by educator Abraham Flexner—sharply divided U.S. medical practice into two incongruent parts: modern medicine, based on physics and chemistry and peer review in scientific journals, and all other forms called "quackery," which lacked scientific proof. Originally, the successes of science were admirable. Surgery conquered new frontiers—for instance, in the chest cavity and in the brain, on tiny vessels and delicate organs like the eye. Advances in pharmacology provided medications for high blood pressure, diabetes, and infectious diseases—ailments that had been untreatable just a few decades before. I still remember how excited my father was about them.

Only slowly did it surface that there was a price for these advances. Side effects were gruesome, as in cancer therapy, and dangerous, as in arthritis medication, or at least annoying and alienating. Antibiotics lost their bite as bacteria developed resistance. People began to feel vulnerable and alone with their fears in the middle of the hectic activity of highly specialized medicine.

Consequently, more and more people have slowly returned to "unscientific" methods and practitioners. They now look in bookstores and libraries for help from traditional and nontraditional new cures. Easy access to the Internet has exploded the quest for better health into gigantic dimensions.

Once belittled as "old wives' tales" and unscientific lore, unfit for the twentieth century's pharmacological advances and surgical heroics, herbs are inspiring public interest in the new millennium. Medicinal herbs are growing ever more popular. Patients are voting with their feet—and their pocketbooks—for medications with fewer side effects. Herbs reconnect you to nature, and you should be leery of a practice of medicine that denies your basic connection with the earth.

Many wonderful books can introduce you to herbs much better than I can do it here. (My favorite is James Duke's *The Green Pharmacy*.) So I will restrict myself here to the discussion of some basic rules and descriptions of some gentle herbs with very high safety records. As it turns out, nearly all the herbs Sebastian Kneipp used fall into this category. He had tried each herb on himself before he prescribed it to patients (I wish modern doctors would do that with their medicines!). More complicated and stronger herbs belong in the hands of specialists.

We are just beginning to finally use *all* therapies—the alternative and the conventional—in an integrative manner to the benefit of everybody. And in the traditional canon of cures, gentle herbs have always been the foundation.

Even when you use herbs only for spice and flavor in the kitchen and in teas, there are numerous health benefits. Medicinal herbs against a variety of health conditions can be sorted in two ways:

1. As *remedies* against diseases, taken in such forms as extracts, tinctures, capsules, and tablets, for either acute conditions (short-term use) or chronic conditions (long-term use).
2. As *tonics* (also called *adaptogens* or *alteratives*) for general strengthening and well-being. Tonics work mainly on the immune system and the endocrine (gland) system.

Herbs have been used to heal since the beginning of time, and humans are not the first and only species to discover their healing properties. Animals have been observed to search out plants when they feel sick. One study showed forty different plants eaten by horses when they are not feeling well. Cats nibble on grass to throw up the hairballs from their stomachs, and every dog owner knows stories about dogs that eat greens. Apes in the wild will find certain healing plants when necessary and are choosy about what they eat, depending on what they need.

It's not surprising then that plants, including herbs, are built from the same basic building blocks as humans and animals: water, carbohydrates, fats, and proteins, thrown in with a few salts and minerals. Plant cells function in ways that are very similar to ours and contain the same tiny cell organelles, including the nucleus with its genetic material of DNA, the mitochondria (the energy factory), and the Golgi apparatus, where proteins are produced. But plants differ from animals and people in one very crucial point: they can't move on their own volition. But even though they cannot move, they still reproduce through flowers and pollination, and they are able to defend themselves against predators such as fungi, bacteria, and viruses in two remarkable ways. They defend themselves against veggie-eating predators by making themselves unpalatable. And they are able to prevent microorganisms (fungi, bacteria, viruses) from invading the plant tissues.

These amazing defenses would not exist without water. Never forget this most basic and sacred element is the most important part of our bodies—and the most important part of plants as well. Without water neither the herbs nor we would be alive. For millions of years, we ate plants, developed on them and with them. What protects the plants against germs also protects us against germs. Our bodies incorporated plant properties to become stronger and healthier.

The very existence of healing herbs is seen by many herbal healers as the working of divine grace, Sebastian Kneipp among them. Once you see herbs and humans intertwined in a sacred connection (as are all living beings of this earth), environmentalism does not sound like a weird ideology, but a logical consequence. Once you are in awe of the intricate interconnections of all living and nonliving nature, you cannot condone any thoughtless destruction of rain forest or native bog or desert or prairie.

CHAPTER 17

CHOOSING AND BUYING HERBAL PRODUCTS

With all the recent hype around herbs, there is great confusion when it comes to selecting and buying herbal products. With little regulation of the U.S. herbal market, the quality of herbal products ranges from wonderful to awful, and few customers are informed enough to make good choices. For example, everybody seems to be using echinacea for a cold these days, but I assure you, many people are not getting what they think they are buying. This chapter gives you the information you need to select and use herbs effectively and safely.

Types of Herbal Products

Foods can be put into categories according to their freshness, and the same is true for herbs. Let's rank herbal preparations, starting with the freshest:

- **Fresh herbs:** These go right from where they grow in your garden or fields into your teapot or on the table. They are powerhouses of strength and best for your health. A warning is necessary, however: depending on plant traits, soil conditions, sunlight, and other climate factors, pollution, and time of harvest, different batches of herbs will differ widely in quality. But as long as fresh herbs are not heavily polluted or contaminated, these are the best herbs you can get.

- **Freshly pressed herbal juices:** These are widely used in Europe. They are especially favored as bitters and tonics. Organic plants are harvested and immediately brought to the factory and processed. Within hours, the pressed juice is bottled and capped. Since it is an expensive process, these highly efficient herbal juices are becoming more difficult to purchase, even in Europe. But they are one of the mainstays of the Sebastian Kneipp therapy. If I ever would buy a juicer, it would be for herbal juices. Stinging nettle is my favorite.
- **Dried herbs:** If you harvest those fresh, good herbs and dry them, something will get lost inevitably. But if the herb is out of season or does not grow in your backyard, dried herbs are the second best. If you are not growing them yourself— and most people don't—look for a reliable source for dried herbs, since not all are equal. Loose dried herbs should not be stored longer than one year. Often you can just follow your nose and your eyes. If herbs look crumbly, dusty, and faded and smell stale, they are not fresh anymore.
- **Herbal tea bags** are a form of dried herbs and, again, they can be of widely different quality. You have no way of knowing whether you got very fresh herbs or purchased the last sweep from the factory floor. It is a question of trust and trying out. Good-quality herbal tea bags might come sealed individually in foil or cellophane; they taste strong—and they come with a price. For common herbs like chamomile or peppermint, you might use at least two tea bags of the supermarket variety for a cup, in order to assure a decent potency of the ingredients.
- **Infusions:** This is just a fancy name for a watery extract or a tea. For an infusion from dried herbs, take as much as you can grab between your thumb and two fingers for a cup. Use boiling water. Root material often has to be simmered for

a time; follow the prescription on the package. Fresh herbs are about ten times heavier (because of the water) than dried material, so you need about a fistful for a cup. Infusions should be used within the day.

- **Extracts:** Alcoholic extracts are made by letting dried or fresh herbs macerate (just sit) in 35 to 90 percent medicinal alcohol. Extracts are never taken directly into the mouth, but are always diluted in water.
- **Nonalcoholic extracts:** Some people do not want to imbibe alcohol, even in small amounts. Nonalcoholic extracts are made by replacing alcohol with the sweetish glycerin. Always dilute them in water.
- **Tinctures:** These are watered-down extracts, but they should still be taken in fluid.
- **Mixtures:** Several tinctures are mixed together for convenience—for instance, in an herbal formula for premenstrual syndrome (PMS). The disadvantage is that if you experience an allergic response, it is difficult to figure out which ingredient caused it. Therefore, I usually prefer single herbs to ready-made concoctions.
- **Inhalations:** Inhalations are usually made from fresh or dried herbs or extracts added to a pot of steaming hot water. The steam is then inhaled with a towel over one's head. Beware of scalding!
- **Capsules:** Herbal capsules are filled with the powder that results when liquid alcoholic extract is freeze-dried. The capsules are often made from gelatin, an animal product that theoretically could contain BSE particles (bovine spongiforme encephalitis, the cause of mad cow disease). Vegetarian capsules also are available. Capsules are easier to take, particularly on the go. But they are down one step on the freshness scale. Capsules containing a concentrated liquid extract are better.
- **Tablets:** Herbal tablets are made by freeze-drying an alcoholic extract and pressing the resulting powder with

other ingredients, often starch or talc, into tablet form. Further ingredients are added for better coherence and for flavor and looks. Because of the extra, unnecessary ingredients and prolonged processing, I avoid tablets.

- **Coated tablets:** Coating tablets requires another processing step to mask bitter or metallic tastes. The more ingredients involved, the more likely it is that one will experience allergies with the end product.

- **Syrups:** Herbal syrups are made of tinctures in a thick sugar base. Most syrups contain high-fructose corn syrup; I discourage their use. But you can make your own syrup from cane sugar at home for children. Be careful with dosage. After taking syrup, brush your teeth.

- **Ointments:** Made by adding herbal extracts to a semisolid base, ointments are often made from petroleum-based agents and are used on the skin. All store-bought ointments and lotions need preservatives, even the ones labeled organic. For home use, lanolin and olive oil make a healthier base, but they need to be kept in the refrigerator.

- **Lotions:** Herbal lotions are more liquid than ointments, made with an alcohol/water mix. The alcohol can be drying for the skin.

- **Enemas and suppositories:** These herbal products are medicines for rectal application. Suppositories are popular in Europe, less so here. Suppositories often have a base combining glycerin, gelatin, lecithin, and oil. Vaginal suppositories also are available.

Choosing a Good Herbal Product

When buying an herbal product, it's difficult to know exactly what you're getting, because routine testing is not done on these products in the United States. The following tips may help you to find better products:

- **Look for products made from fresh, organically grown plants.** Organic products are hardier because they are not pampered and protected by pesticides and herbicides, so they contain more active ingredients. And they are less contaminated. Of course, nowadays it is impossible to be completely free from pollutants; there always will be some airborne contamination or pollution of water and soil.

- **Look for the companies that manufacture, store, and ship properly.** Herbs, like fresh food, need to be shipped and stored under optimal temperatures. The final product you find in your health food store cannot be better than the original plant in the field or the wild. And while it is harvested, shipped, stored, sieved, ground, and further processed, it loses freshness and potency fast. A big, reputable firm has a name to lose and will adhere better to standards.

- **Pay attention to the active ingredients.** Patenting laws are such that one cannot patent a whole plant, but one can patent a concoction that is made from single substances derived from a plant—the famous aspirin example. This is why you will find tons of commercial products that claim they used the most active substance(s) for their special product. Mistrust those claims! Try to find a local healer and plant gatherer. She might provide you with a cheap, whole product.

- **If you're not using fresh herbs, look for products that are standardized.** To be sure that the manufacturer is following proper standards, look for United States Pharmacopeia (USP) or National Formulary (NF) on the label. Standardized herbs usually come from a respectable firm, but standardization also has its drawbacks. The ingredient the product is standardized to might not be the most active ingredient. Also, standardization requires more mixing, diluting, and enhancing, so it involves more processing. If I dry my own herbs at home, I know they are not adulterated. So while standardization gives you a certain protection from fraud, it doesn't necessarily give you a better product—and definitely not a cheaper product. However, if you're not in a position to grow your own herbs, look for products that are standardized.

- **Do your homework before you buy herbs.** Investigate which herbs are best for specific health conditions, and learn how to read the labels. Have a physician recommend them, or use books and the Internet, but always beware that many sellers do not have your health, but only their purses, in mind. U.S. labeling laws don't allow manufacturers to tell you exactly what an herbal product may do for you. Sellers may not make claims about specific conditions, but they may make more general statements about wellness. For example, the label of an herbal product may not say, "This is for bronchitis," but a manufacturer may tell you that a product might be good for the lungs. Therefore, you usually have to inform yourself about what you need before you buy your herbs. Always buy from the best source available—not from the cheapest. Also, because herbs are treated as foods by law, manufacturers do not mention possible side effects. A good herbal preparation should have information available on the label that tells you what it contains, which ingredient(s) or fraction it was standardized to, the expiration date, and possibly the state or country of origin. The label also should list the daily dosage and storage requirements.

Taking the Correct Dosages

Always check with your doctor before taking any herbs! Then follow the recommendations on the bottle or the package. For acute diseases (short-term conditions, such as a cold), take the highest recommended dosage, not longer than two weeks. For chronic diseases, take the lowest recommended dosage. Herbs usually act more slowly and mildly than conventional drugs, so for a chronic disease, you might have to take herbs for months before you see a result. Some herbs should not be taken that long; discuss this with your doctor.

Sometimes an option for chronic conditions is to rotate herbs that have similar effects. After three to four weeks, you might stop taking a particular herb for three to four weeks (unless your doctor says differently) and instead take another herb that has similar properties. You could continue in the same way with a third, and so on.

Children do well with herbs generally, but you cannot assume that all herbs are safe for children. Consult your pediatric doctor. At the other end of the age span, because elderly people experience decreasing kidney function, they should use herbs with caution, especially root herbs. Pregnant women should not take any herb without consulting with her obstetrician. Even kitchen herbs should be used sparingly.

Botanical Safety Guidelines

Many herbs are safe and beneficial if you observe these safety guidelines:

- Don't use herbs while you are pregnant.
- Don't take herbs while you are breast-feeding.
- Take herbs only after discussing them with a conventional doctor who is up-to-date on the healing powers of herbs.
- Before taking herbs that are unsafe—foxglove, comfrey (internally), pennyroyal, and others—get advice from a specialist. The salesperson in the store is *not* a specialist; always ask your doctor.
- Before you try herbs, if you are also taking conventional drugs (such as Coumadin), discuss possible interactions with your pharmacist and doctor.
- Never take herbs from dubious or polluted sources.

HERBS FROM THE OCEAN:
SEAWEEDS AND ALGAE

Seaweeds and algae are healing herbs from the ocean. Seaweeds are high in calcium and other minerals but also relatively high in sodium, so they should never be eaten in large amounts. In addition, they are a good source of iodine, which can be a problem for overactive thyroid conditions. Sprinkle them over salads and into stews and soups, and have them as snacks in small pieces. Sushi, for example, is often wrapped in nori, a type of seaweed.

The following common forms of seaweed and algae are among the edible varieties:

- Kelp
- Dulse
- Hijiki (or hiziki)
- Nori (or laver)
- Kombu
- Alaria

Herbal Teas: The Best Medicine

Tea is the most favored form of herbal preparation and not just for historical and nostalgic reasons. A tea from freshly gathered herbs is the most effective way to get the healing power out of a plant. In a watery extract (that's a tea), you get between 50 and 90 percent of the effective ingredients. Tea from fresh plants contains a few more effective ingredients than are present even in dried plants. But a medicinal tea from dried herbs is still a very good source, provided the plants are not older than one year or are kept fresh in an airtight package.

Some plant compounds, especially those found in roots, are not dissolved by water. They need to be extracted with alcohol. Echinacea is an example. A watery solution will not help your immune system much. Not even the chopped-up, above-the-ground parts of the plants will do, but only an alcoholic extract of the roots.

But overall, a tea is the ideal vehicle to get the best value from an herb. A tea is cheap, easy to use, and effective. It fills the body with warm fluid. And the time it takes to prepare and drink the tea gives you a respite from stress and hectic activity—something that popping a pill cannot give you.

Making your own herbal tea is easy and a very effective way to help heal a variety of health problems. In the next chapter, you'll find out how to brew your own herbal tea, as well as how to use many healing herbs and spices in the kitchen to improve your health and well-being.

CHAPTER 18

HEALING HERBS AND SPICES IN THE KITCHEN

Kitchen herbs spice up bland dishes and give the extra bonus of promoting health. As we've seen, herbs can be grown in the garden, and it is a marvelous hobby. Some herbs will even thrive on the windowsill; many a gardener started out in that small way. Here are a few herbs that you might want to consider using in your kitchen:

- Arugula
- Basil
- Borage
- Burnet
- Chamomile flowers
- Chives
- Cilantro
- Dill
- Fennel
- Lemon balm
- Marjoram
- Oregano
- Parsley
- Peppermint and other mints
- Red clover
- Rosemary
- Sage
- Savory
- Thyme
- Watercress

Spices That Promote Health

Spices, like herbs, give flavor to your food and are loaded with antioxidants. They also prevent food from spoiling—one reason why hot climates often have hot cuisines. In kitchen terms, the word *herbs* usually refers to green herbs (fresh or dried), whereas *spices* are often made from the dried, ground fruits, roots or bark of plants and are usually more pungent than herbs. The distinction between spices and herbs is not always exact. Here are some examples of spices:

- Allspice
- Bay leaf
- Black pepper
- Caraway
- Cardamom
- Cayenne
- Cinnamon
- Cloves

- Curry
- Fenugreek
- Ginger
- Nutmeg
- Paprika
- Turmeric
- Vanilla

How to Grow and Brew Your Own Garden Tea

A fresh herbal tea can be invigorating. If you like to grow things, try to create a small herb garden, either in your backyard or on a bright windowsill. Making your own tea from plants that you have grown and gathered is both satisfying and reassuring: you know what you are getting! I recommend starting with kitchen herbs. Thriving in nearly every soil, they are simple to grow. Sage, chives, thyme, rosemary, oregano, mints, and lemon balm are old standbys. The fun will begin when you go out and harvest from your own garden and beyond—when you bring herbs and edible weeds back from walks.

During the growing season, part of my morning ritual is to go outside and gather a fat handful of herbs for my tea. This reconnects me to nature and gives me some quiet, contemplative time before I start my day. But even if you don't have the luxury of your own garden, you can still make a wonderful tea.

To make your tea, pick a combination of herbs and vegetables. **To avoid potentially poisonous plants, never put something in your mouth that you have not identified 100 percent; 99 percent is not good enough!** When in doubt, throw it out. Don't assume that all parts of a plant are edible because one part is. For instance, while a fresh tomato is delicious, the leaves of the tomato plant are poisonous. Books and the Internet can help you to identify plants. You might also enroll in a botanical course or go on a local field trip.

If you pick from clean sites and haven't sprayed your roses with unmentionable pesticides, you don't need to wash your herbs. In fact, new studies suggest that a little bit of soil and dirt will strengthen your immune system. But make yourself knowledgeable about local wildlife diseases before your harvest.

After you have gathered your big handful of herbs, put them in a pot or coffee press, and pour boiling water over them. A glass pot shows off the green beauty of your herbs. Let them steep for a few minutes. Keep them on a warmer, and enjoy your tea all day long. There is enough taste and green life force left in the plants for steeping them several additional times.

If you like, you may add any kitchen herbs and vegetables that you are growing, as well as raw plant material from your refrigerator: herbs, lettuce, other vegetables, or fruit. Raisins lend sweetness. Your tea will taste very interesting—and different every time, because the ingredients will change with the seasons. If you already drink green tea and like it, you'll be ecstatic about the smooth, rich flavor of your herbal tea.

CAUTION: Always check herbs with your doctor before taking them, especially if you also take conventional medicines. Never use any herb that you have not identified 100 percent.

Some Edible (and Drinkable) Herbs and Plants to Use in Your Teas

- Birch leaves
- Blackberry leaves
- Calendula petals
- Carnation flowers
- Cherry and other stone fruit blossoms (not the leaves)
- Chicory flowers and buds
- Citrus blossoms (lemon, orange, grapefruit, etc.)
- Cornflower or bachelor's button flowers
- Dandelion flowers and leaves
- Echinacea flowers and leaves
- English daisies whole plants
- Feverfew flowers and leaves
- Forsythia flowers
- Goldenrod flowers and upper leaves
- Good King Henry
- Hollyhock flowers
- Honeysuckle flowers
- Jade plant
- Johnny-jump-up flowers and leaves
- Kudzu flowers and leaves
- Lavender blossoms and leaves
- Lilac flowers
- Linden flowers
- Marshmallow flowers
- Nasturtium flowers, buds, leaves, seedpods
- Pansy flowers and leaves
- Petunia flowers
- Plantain leaves
- Purslane leaves
- Raspberry leaves
- Rose petals and leaves and rose hips
- Snapdragon flowers

- Sorrel leaves
- Stinging nettle leaves
- Violet flowers and leaves
- Wild strawberry flowers and leaves

Herbs for Specific Health Issues

Some of our most common health problems can be alleviated with herbal remedies. This section provides ideas for addressing specific problems. But in any situation, be sure to consult a doctor before you try these suggestions.

Herbs to Use in Teas for Your Mind

Herbal teas can be soothing, refreshing, and help with memory or anxiety. Always consult with your physician.

- Ginkgo—against memory loss
- Ginseng—for strengthening the mind (after age fifty) (American ginseng is preferred even by the Chinese. Stop if you get heart palpitations.)
- Hops—for sleep
- Saint-John's-wort—against mild to moderate depression; may induce photosensitivity (a skin rash on sun exposure) and may interfere with certain conventional medications
- Kava kava—against anxiety (Kava has been linked to liver damage). Take it sparingly, and not in conjunction with alcohol, Tylenol (acetaminophen), and other liver-toxic pills).
- Lemon balm—for calming
- Passionflower—for sleep
- Skullcap—for relaxation
- Valerian—for calming and for sleep (It has a distinct taste that some people don't like.)

Herbs Against the Common Cold

I always keep these four herbal extracts in my refrigerator and take them at the first signs of a cold:

- Echinacea
- Pau d'arco
- Osha (*Ligusticum porteri*, also called Indian root or bear medicine, has antiviral properties and works especially well on the respiratory system.)
- Olive leaf extract

Take them three or four times a day according to the label in hot water. If you get worse with them, see your physician. Don't take them longer than two weeks, since a normal cold should be gone by then.

CAUTION: Echinacea should not be taken if you have an autoimmune disease such as multiple sclerosis.

DR. ALEXA'S COUGH TEA

If you have a cough, put the following ingredients into a big mug. Add boiling water, and steep for a few minutes. Drink this three times a day, not more than a week.

I teaspoon dried peppermint leaves
I teaspoon honeysuckle flowers
½ teaspoon dried, ground ginger (or I teaspoon chopped fresh gingerroot)
2 to 3 cloves
I dropperful horehound extract

Aromatherapy for Sleep

Herbs for aromatherapy would be the first step I would try for insomnia because it is the least intrusive method. Bring a drop of essential oil onto an aromatherapy terra-cotta ring that goes over a lightbulb. The hot lightbulb will disperse the oil in the room. Soothing music will enhance the effect. The following herbs are associated with sound, restful sleep:

- Sage
- Sandalwood
- Clary

Herbs for Sleep

As for herbs to be taken by mouth, commercial mixtures of some of these herbs are available. They are convenient. But if you get an allergy, you won't know what the culprit is. Make sure you read the chapter about sleeplessness first because sleep hygiene might be a better way to deal with the problem. Anyway, these herbs, taken in moderation, certainly beat stronger medications. But even with herbs, you can get dependent. Therefore I prefer to take them singly and to rotate them.

- Hops
- Passionflower
- Valerian
- Skullcap
- Chamomile
- Lemon balm

Menopausal Herbs

Menopause can be a taxing time in a woman's life with hot flashes, mood swings, sleeplessness, crawling of the legs, vaginal dryness, urinary tract symptoms, headaches, fatigue, and the erratic menstrual cycle: too short, too long, too heavy, too scant, and not at all. You certainly need the advice of an experienced gynecological specialist. But if she explains that this is all just normal, you can try this mixture:

- Black cohosh
- Red clover
- Wild yam
- Ginkgo biloba

You might want to start with these herbs twice a day, and reduce it to once a day as soon as you feel better.

CAUTION: These herbs should not be taken if your estrogen is still high or if you have breast or ovarian cancer or take Coumadin.

Herbs for Your Gums

For sensitive and bleeding gums or deep pockets, brush, floss, and use a dental water jet. In addition, use the following herbs:

- Tea tree oil: Mix one drop in half a glass of water; rinse mouth.
- Myrrh tincture: Mix a few drops in half a glass of water; rinse mouth.
- Aloe vera: Scrape out the inside gel of an aloe leaf (about a teaspoonful), and chew it. Then swallow: it is also good for your stomach.

Herbs for Your Organs

The following herbs may help you with an assortment of ailments. Always check with your doctor first.

- Saw palmetto berries—for the prostate
- Tea tree oil—applied to your skin to treat wounds and fungus
- Chamomile—for your stomach
- Milk thistle—for your liver
- Arnica cream—to treat bruises externally—do not swallow (only for unbroken skin)
- Hawthorn—for your heart

Herbs for Calcium and Bone Health

Strong bones need more than calcium. All plants provide balanced food for your bones. But here are some herbs that have been researched and found especially potent against osteoporosis:

- Basil
- Black pepper
- Celery seed
- Chervil
- Cinnamon
- Dandelion
- Dill weed
- Fennel
- Fenugreek
- Ginseng
- Licorice
- Marjoram
- Oregano
- Parsley
- Pigweed
- Poppy seed
- Purslane
- Red clover
- Sage
- Savory
- Seaweeds (especially kelp)
- Stinging nettle
- Thyme
- Watercress

Herbs as Tonics and Adaptogens

The herbs we have talked about so far address specific conditions and diseases. Tonics (also called adaptogens or alteratives—an old word meaning "altering your state") on the other hand, improve overall health without a specific target, but they may work mostly on the immune and endocrine systems. They are taken over a longer time period than the usual disease-specific herbs mentioned previously. They have an overall invigorating effect. Read the label, and stay at the lowest recommended dose.

Pick and choose from the list below—only take one or two herbs at a time. Some can be used in the kitchen. Mushrooms all seem to have an invigorating effect on the immune system; therefore, I use them nearly daily in my stir-fry dishes. Never eat mushrooms raw—they are toxic.

- Ashwaganda
- Asian or American ginseng
- Astragalus
- Eleuthero
- Garlic
- Ginger
- Holy basil
- Licorice
- Maitake mushroom
- Reishi mushroom
- Rhodiola
- Schisandra
- Siberian ginseng
- Stinging nettle

PART 5

LIFE BALANCE

FOLLOWING
NATURE'S RHYTHMS

NOTHING IS MORE SOOTHING AND RELAXING THAN A DAY AT the beach. At the beach, you give in and let things happen. You don't fight the tide; you go with the flow. You are naturally attuned to the rhythms of the powerful ocean, the rejuvenating wind, the soothing sameness of the waves. A natural order, or rhythm, governs the world, an order as inexorable as the ebb and flow of waves on an ocean beach. You are part of this rhythm too because you are from the ocean and carry the ocean tides within. The monthly rhythm of the moon pulls on your body too—yes, even if you are male. Nothing you can do will alter this eternal rhythm, and you have to go with the flow of this rhythm to ensure your maximum health and well-being, both physical and mental. Besides being a bag full of water that reacts to the moon's gravity, you can learn more from ebb and flow. There are tides in your life too: ups and downs, inevitable phases as you age, tides of your well-being, peaks and troughs of your career and your moods—it is time to learn from ebb and flow.

If only you could incorporate that natural rhythm into your daily life! The wave of the ocean is as much a metaphor as your internal reality. Because the tides of the oceans are governed by the moon, your internal rhythms are too. They are obvious in the female rhythms of menstruation that come every twenty-eight days, and less obvious in, for instance, sleep patterns that change with the ascent and descent of the moon. Science is just at the beginning of discovering these ancient rhythms of our physiology—and how modern life, so rhythm-deaf, hurts our health, our moods, and even the next generations.

The rhythm of the ocean is regular but by no means mechanical. The tides come higher or lower with the phases of the moon, weather stirs up the waters, and storms rip across the sea. But through all that, the steady rhythm of the ocean stays the same. As not a single drop of water in the world gets lost, the life (and actions) of every human being resonates everywhere. The wisdom of water will help you achieve the quiet joy of order from childhood into old age. Even in the nineteenth century, Sebastian Kneipp realized that you cannot be healthy if you live against the grain, if you live against nature. Modern life has separated us from nature, and health problems are the result.

CHAPTER 19

THE TIDES WITHIN US

Keeping with Your Natural Rhythms

The prescription is easy: you must become sensitive to the rhythms in nature and not go against them if you want to remain strong and healthy. Unfortunately, following this prescription is not so easy in our modern, hectic, hyperalarmed world. But you could try some simple things like sleeping before midnight, fasting between dinner and breakfast, and eating seasonal food—and see how much better you feel. There is a long list of health problems that result from disturbing the natural life rhythms. Science has already investigated the negative effects of disruptions to our circadian rhythms that result from working the night shift, jet lag, and not sleeping in total darkness. If you observe yourself and others, you will see that your body, mind, and emotions change with the seasons, the time of the month, and, of course, the time of day. But when was the last time you consciously sat down at dusk on a bench to observe the setting sun and listen to the birds' evening songs?

The solution of personal, medical, and even societal problems might be closer if we understand ourselves in the context of nature and see ourselves as a part of all life on the planet. Anybody who gardens becomes aware that all beauty finally ends up in the compost pile: a humbling and refreshing view of life. Modern times have removed us from our ancient rhythms. Many people think nothing of going grocery shopping at three o'clock in the morning, eating fresh oranges and strawberries when winter has covered the fields with heavy snow, flying to Florida to escape the cold and going skiing far into summer, skipping breakfast and having a huge dinner late in the night, overheating rooms in the middle of winter, and flying through several time zones in one day and expecting to arrive fresh for a full program of work or sightseeing. Saddest of all is when we barely notice the first smell of early spring because we are so connected to telephone, computer, and television.

Connect with Nature and Soil

No life is a full life if it lacks the contact with nature and the soil. When we lose that connection, we lose ourselves and our purpose (not to mention that we might destroy the earth in the process). I believe in daily walks—as much as possible in some green space. Gardening is a wonderful way to connect with nature, if only on your windowsill or your balcony (try growing some of the herbs described in this book). Look at the sky and smell the air. Watch the sun come up and go down whenever possible.

What it does: Reconnects you to what is important in life, in you.

Time required: Every minute spent in your garden or outdoors is bliss.

Props needed: Soil and gardening tools; determination to find a park if you live in an urban environment.

Cautions: None.

Touch: A Hug a Day

Touch is important for well-being. Humans lived for millions of years in tribes and large families. At night, our ancestors slept in one big pile, rolled in with people and bearskins. Touch was common. Now children of ten learn that all touch is sexual and dangerous. Many of us live in one-person households and work in separate cubicles without daily touch, and this loneliness makes us prone to depression, violence, and infections. So try to hug someone every day (not against someone's will, of course!).

What it does: Restores a sense of well-being to the hugger and the hugged.

Time required: Seconds.

Props needed: None.

Caution: In times of flu epidemics, avoid hugging. But people who do hug get much fewer infections—probably because of decreased stress hormones. (And, indeed, some kinds of touch can be inappropriate.)

The Importance of Balance

Balance in all you do—work and play, activity and sleep—is essential in your everyday life for you to feel replenished, not exhausted. You can create balance in your life by reintroducing yourself to the natural order that keeps you in sync with the internal patterns and rhythms of your body and mind.

Do you feel exhausted? If you are like millions of other people, chances are that you do. You might find that you are getting sick more often than you used to. You might either be unable to sleep or want to sleep all the time. Your house might look like a bomb exploded in it. You might have anxiety or difficulty concentrating; and you might have lost the simple joy in life that you once had as your birthright. These symptoms may arise from not living according to your body's natural rhythms.

For example, when was the last time you watched a sunrise? When I was a child, my father would often bundle me up in blankets and take me out at dawn to watch. That early in the morning, the air and the light have a quality that is beneficial to our well-being. Overnight, the air has been replenished with oxygen by the trees and been blown clean by the wind to the very middle of the city, and fresh air lets the radiance of the light give the new day its shine. Filling your lungs with deep breaths at this time of the day will fill the rest of your day with replenishing oxygen.

In the evening, do you wind down when the dusk sinks over the land, or do you have to squeeze in another party, another household chore, another hour of TV with upsetting news? Or could you take the time for a walk with a friend, a child, a spouse to see the sun setting or stare into the fire for a while, doing nothing?

Taking time out of every day to appreciate the rhythm of just day and night will reinstate some of our mental, emotional, and physical well-being.

HEALTH$_2$O BALANCE

Your qi (pronounced *chi*), or life energy, is limited. Learn to:

- Use Earth's resources—water, fresh air, unspoiled wilderness—responsibly.
- Safeguard your energy and put it to good work on worthwhile causes; don't waste it.
- Be grateful for little pleasures.
- Avoid toxins like sugars, smoking, recreational drugs, and alcohol.
- Practice moderation in eating, acquisitions, and using up Earth's resources.
- Practice kindness and "nonharming" toward your fellow travelers and all creatures.

- Make use of unspoiled nature around you with walking and hiking.
- Let go of envy and old grievances; practice forgiveness.
- Honor family, friendships, and places.
- Strengthen your immune system with cold water every day.
- Take every opportunity to move because movement makes you happy.
- Nourish your body with fresh foods preferably from local sources.
- Use herbs freely in the kitchen and for ailments.

Ebb and flow are as natural and unavoidable in your life as they are on Earth. Try to find balance in the tides of your life in:

- Work and play
- Activity and relaxation
- Effort and sleep
- Honoring traditions and learning new tricks
- Maintaining your standpoint and practicing tolerance
- Helping others and taking time for self-fulfillment.
- Staying young and acknowledging aging

CHAPTER 20

RESTORING LIFE BALANCE TO HEAL COMMON HEALTH PROBLEMS

M any common health problems are related to disturbances in our natural bodily rhythms. This chapter identifies some of the frequent complaints I hear from my patients and offers suggestions for restoring balance.

Common Cold

A daily cold shower after your warm one (described in Chapter 4) will build up your immune system to ward off colds and flu. A cold shower certainly reduces the frequency of colds but might not eliminate them totally. If you feel yourself coming down with something, use the saltwater nose rinse (described in Chapter 6) several times a day. Herbal remedies are described in Chapter 18 and can be also used against the flu. In addition, these practices can help you recover from a cold:

- Rest. Your body is trying to tell you something. To get sick, it takes two: a virus and a run-down immune system. Get out of your hectic schedule as soon as you feel the first little itch in your nose, the first scratch in your throat, or the first heaviness in your muscles. You know when you do not feel all right. Go to sleep immediately when you come home—or right after you have implemented the following measures.

- Take a warm to hot footbath, followed by a cold gush.
- Use steam inhalation, along with herbs. (See Chapter 18 for recommendations.)
- If you do not have a fever, a warm bath with herbs may help. (Use eucalyptus, pine and other evergreens, or thyme.)
- Make some hot blueberry soup. Barely cover the contents of one package of frozen blueberries from the supermarket with water; bring to a fast boil. Then slowly eat the berries and liquid. This soup contains vitamins and minerals to help fight infection, and the blue color in the blueberries kills infectious agents, too. (By the way, blueberry soup is also good for acute stomach flu and urinary tract infections.)
- Avoid over-the-counter cold medications. They alleviate the symptoms but hinder the immune system from healing your body. They might increase the clogging by drying the sinus contents, and they lower your temperature when your body is trying to produce a fever to kill the germs.
- Linden flowers or elderflowers as a hot tea will induce sweating and healing. Drink it in tiny sips as hot as possible and very slowly to prolong the contact with the mucosa of your throat. The idea is to keep stimulating blood flow to your throat.

Constipation

It is interesting that people talk about their digestive problems with the term *regularity*, because regularity—that is, order—is the answer to the problem. You eat and you eliminate; those are the basic physiological functions that keep us alive. When the elimination function is blocked, it is called constipation. This is usually thought to be a disease that needs to be treated with pills (laxatives). In reality, constipation is a poor function of an organ as it interacts with our environment (the food we eat). It is not a disease—but it can lead to diseases—and laxatives are not the answer. The exercise, water, and nutrition recommendations earlier in this book are essential for good bowel health. In addition, I recommend the following practices to relieve constipation:

- Drink seven glasses of water, preferably warm, each day. Drink more if the weather is hot or you are exercising.
- Never suppress the urge to move your bowels. The longer these undesirable substances linger inside you, the more likely cancer and reabsorption of toxins become. Also, if you override the urge, the stool thickens and gets harder to expel.
- Avoid antibiotics (except, of course, in life-threatening situations when antibiotics are necessary) because they destroy the healthful bowel bacteria. Take probiotics daily, usually acidophilus, bifidus, and benign *E. coli* populations; they build up a healthy bowel flora. You find probiotics in the fridge section of your health food store.
- Digestion starts with chewing well, and if everything you eat is soft, the digestion process does not function well from the beginning. There is a saying in German pertaining to food: soft in, hard out; hard in, soft out. So give your teeth some work to do.

Here are some gentle herb and food remedies for constipation:

- Prunes
- Unsweetened prune juice
- Flaxseed (thoroughly chewed or freshly ground is better than store-bought ground)
- Psyllium

- Ginger
- Fenugreek
- Garlic
- Sweet violets
- Apple

The old saying "An apple a day keeps the doctor away" might well stem from the laxative benefits of apples.

High Blood Pressure (Hypertension)

About 5 percent of high-blood-pressure cases turn out to be caused by a real disease (usually kidney disease, endocrine conditions, or tumors). However, the other 95 percent are related to lifestyle. Fifty percent of all Americans will be diagnosed with hypertension at one point in their lives. Since high blood pressure is mainly a self-inflicted disease, it is the perfect reason to bring *order* and rhythm back into your life.

High blood pressure has mainly two causes. Circulating stress hormones drive the heart to work too hard, and too much salt in the system increases the water pressure in the blood vessels. And as constant hard words in a marriage lead to a hardening of all the tender feelings in the relationship, so does constant high blood pressure lead to hardening of the arteries. Stiff arteries cannot respond well to changes in demand, and they might rupture, just as high water pressure in the pipes may burst the plumbing. Heart disease, stroke, kidney failure, and impotence are the most common effects of long-term hypertension.

Reducing high blood pressure can be as simple as following the guidelines in this book, especially those about cold showers, cold arm baths, daily exercise (start with two minutes a day, as described in Chapter 9), and focusing your diet on fresh vegetables and fruits, while avoiding sodium, white flour and white sugar, dairy, and bad fats. And drink enough water to flush out dangerous salts.

Insomnia: Restore Your Natural Sleep Rhythm

Tiredness is relative: If you step over your natural point of sleepiness in the evening, you get a second wind (well known to doctors from residency times), and you can go on for a few hours more. That is why, after your favorite TV show ends and you are ready to go to sleep, you might find yourself sitting upright in bed, unable to let go and sleep. Then you will show up at the doctor's office to complain about insomnia and ask for a sleeping pill. I call insomnia the curse of our times, the human cost of harnessing electricity. A sleeping pill, also called a "hypnotic sedative," will change your sleep patterns by disturbing your natural brain waves, inducing a quasi sleep that is less refreshing than natural sleep, and might leave you with a hangover and an addiction to sleeping pills. (For occasional, more benign help with sleeping, please see the section on herbs and aromatherapy. But I first recommend following the sleep hygiene suggestions in this chapter.)

For most people, a natural lull happens in their energy around 9:00 to 9:30 P.M., when their bodies want to go to sleep (for some, it might happen as early as 6:00 P.M.). This is our ancient heritage: the campfire has burned down, and the tribe hits the bearskins. But because of watching TV, partying late, working overtime, playing computer games, or eating after dinner, we override our body's signals for sleep. As a resident, I had to get over my sleeping point many, many times. It is possible. But it is not healthy.

In addition to the relaxing herbal and aromatherapy remedies described in Chapter 18, here are some other suggestions for restoring your natural sleep rhythm:

- Make sure your bedroom is quiet and as dark as possible.
  Even a small amount of light while you sleep disrupts the
  production of melatonin, an important sleep hormone. It is
  also a good idea to teach your children early that darkness is
  nothing to fear instead of installing a night-light.
- During the day, make sure you get enough exercise (see the
  ideas in Part 2) and enough exposure to bright daytime light.

In the evening, begin to dim the lights in your house to encourage the production of melatonin, a sleep hormone.

- If you have worries, write them down in a journal. Then read something soothing to empty your mind of your worries.
- Avoid late-night meals; don't eat after dinner.
- Sleep on a firm mattress with your window open whenever possible. Most of the time, indoor pollution is worse than outdoor pollution. Sleep in the nude to allow your skin to breathe and detoxify your body. I like a soft flannel sheet close to my body.
- Avoid caffeine and chocolate if you are having trouble sleeping.
- Before you go to sleep, read something pleasant, listen to soothing music, meditate, or try the evening breathing exercise (see Chapter 13).
- Wet socks (see Chapter 8) are fabulous against insomnia.
- Keep a dream journal at your bedside. If you wake up in the middle of the night, use the time to try to understand the meaning of your dreams.
- Don't use alcohol as a sleeping aid. Alcohol helps you fall asleep because it dulls brain function. But as soon as it wears off, your brain will be in a state of excitement, and you will wake up prematurely. Tranquilizers and sleeping pills might have a similar effect.
- Talk to your physician about any medical problems, such as pain, that are keeping you awake, as well as the sleep-robbing effects of many prescription and over-the-counter drugs.

CHAPTER 21

PUTTING IT ALL TOGETHER

THE FIVE WATER ESSENTIALS

IN ACTION

Any of the Five Water Essentials help you to get the most out of each day of your life. Thus, they double as motivational tools. If you take a cold shower in the morning, you feel so good that you want to do more for your health during the day—perhaps by following your shower with some yoga or meditation. If you go for a ten-minute walk before lunch, you return to the cafeteria with a refocused sense of healthy nutrition, and you might even go for another ten-minute walk after lunch. Your wholesome lunch makes you less prone to that infamous after-lunch sag, and if you feel yourself losing your posture at your computer, you immediately want to get out of that slump with micromovements or a yoga posture.

In the evening, instead of just collapsing on your sofa or being grouchy with the kids, you run for just two minutes on your treadmill or retire into your quiet corner for five minutes of meditation. Thus you unwind faster and return to a tired but relaxed balance, creating an evening filled with the joy and leisure that comes from a day well done and intensively lived. Going to bed by nine o'clock, definitely before ten, will let you look forward to a new day instead of dreading the alarm clock.

Your Health-by-Water Invigorating Day

Here is a sample of a day filled with the Five Water Essentials. Throughout your sample day, you'll do exercises and procedures that are easy and often look like nothing, but you will notice a difference in the way you feel physically and mentally when you're finished. Start on a weekend so you'll have the leisure to read up on things you have forgotten and see how the practice fits into your schedule.

Step 1   Do morning breathing and micro movements before getting out of bed (2–4 minutes).

Step 2   Get up to see the sun rise; connect with your spiritual nature (1 minute).

Step 3   Take a cold shower (1 minute) or cold wash (2 minutes).

Step 4   Stand on one leg while brushing your teeth (no extra time).

Step 5   Do a nose rinse (1 minute).

Step 6   Do one yoga stance of your choice (5 minutes).

Step 7   Eat breakfast: leftovers from dinner or balanced carbohydrates, fats, and protein with some fresh fruit. Sit down for it (30 minutes).

Step 8   Try to walk to work. At least plan to walk 10 minutes per day. Park the car far away. Always use the stairs instead of the escalator and elevator (10 minutes, accumulated throughout the day).

Step 9   Do micro movements (in the car or on public transportation) (no extra time).

Step 10 Sing along in the car with the radio; sing and hum as much as possible (no extra time).

Step 11   Enjoy a 5-minute meditation any time you need it, at
           work or at home—or in your parked car (motor off!).
           It eases the transition from work to home (5 minutes).

Step 12   Take 3 deep breaths and stretch, whenever you use the
           bathroom (no extra time). Splash your face with cold
           water.

Step 13   Lunch on something healthful, such as a pita bread, lean
           meat or chicken, and salad (*without* cheese, deli meats,
           bacon crumbles, or heavy dressing) (no extra time).

Step 14   For dinner eat vegetables, vegetables, vegetables with
           fish or a little meat and a salad (30 to 60 minutes).

Step 15   Write brief notes about your day in your journal.
           Remember to be kind to yourself (5 minutes).

Step 16   Do micro movements as you sit in front of the TV or
           when reading, knitting, or listening to music—whatever
           your recreational activities are (no extra time).

Step 17   Take a cold shower or cold wash (1 minute).

Step 18   Do another nose rinse (1 minute).

Step 19   Do evening breathing (5 minutes).

Step 20   Sleep with your window open (no extra time).

Step 21   Sleep long enough; be in bed by 10 o'clock at least 4
           times a week.

Your Invigorating Week

In addition to your daily routine, build some of the following
suggestions into your weekly routine:

- One class pertaining to your health: a cooking course, a yoga class, or something new that excites you.
- One routine health session, such as a weekly meditation group, a visit to a massage therapist, a few hours in a sauna, or a luxurious hour in your home spa.
- One weekend outing such as taking a long nature walk or hike, going to a swimming pool, horseback riding, visiting a famous garden or outdoor museum, or playing hoops with the kids.
- One extensive grooming session: Take an evening or a couple of hours during the day when you pamper yourself. Give yourself a total-body oil bath.

A FINAL WORD
CONSERVING THE EARTH'S WATER

As a child, I read a story that planted the importance of water in my young mind. It was called "Rainmaker Gertrud," by Theodor Storm. Andrees, the son of a poor widow, is in love with the rich farmer's daughter Maren, but her father objects to their wedding because a desperate drought lies over the land. The young man has to solve the impossible task of making it rain; otherwise he will not get the girl. The drought, while real, is only an excuse; the rich farmer does not want to give his daughter to a poor man. But still, the soil is scorched, the air sizzles, and the cattle perish in the burnt meadows. The birds have ceased to sing.

Eventually, Andrees finds out what he has to do to make it rain: He must wake up Rainmaker Gertrud, who obviously has fallen asleep. And while Rainmaker Gertrud is sleeping, the Fire Devil rules the land. But to find Gertrud's house is an arduous and dangerous task, because the Fire Devil will use every evil trick to prevent Andrees from waking her up.

As it goes in fairy tales, all ends happily for Maren and Andrees. But I remember how the description of the dead silence that lay over the parched land gripped me as a child. Growing up in Hamburg, Germany, where it rains as much as in Oregon, surely hadn't alerted me to the importance of water. But this story did. Without water, there is no life. That insight came back to me, powerfully, with an incident many years ago in Turkey:

Two young Americans and a Turk stood at a tiny stream of water in a vast land of rolling hills covered in brown, dried brush and ochre dirt. The Americans, their feet in a muddy puddle, were shampooing their hair. From between their toes the foamy water dribbled down the hill. The Turk, an older man, pointed to their feet and muttered something in Turkish, which neither the Americans nor I, happening upon the scene, could understand. But I did understand the urgency in his eyes and his gestures down into the valley: the young people were rinsing their hair into the only water source of the man's village.

On March 22, 2005, the United Nations launched its Decade of Water to increase awareness about Earth's dire water situation. The theme is "Water for Life." After you read this book you know how much our health depends on water.

But Earth's waters are in jeopardy. Only about 1 percent of its freshwater is available for us, yet even this is being rapidly rendered unusable. Damming, mining, aqua-farming, and run-off from fertilizers and pesticides pollute rivers and ground-water. Deserts are expanding; loss of vegetation and valuable topsoil is the consequence. Lack of irrigation water in some areas propels huge populations from the country into the cities; overirrigation in other areas empties reservoirs and pulls salts to the surface, thereby rendering soil unusable for crops. Poor water sanitation (meaning no separation between places to collect drinking water and to dump human waste) kills two million children every year. Waterborne diseases, flooding, and tsunamis lead to disasters. Poor wastewater and storm water management makes the water of even water-rich nations expensive and often unpalatable.

Increasingly, water is becoming a political threat. Immigration pressure from dry countries to water-rich Europe and North America is growing. In the United States, interstate rivalries have flared up about the use of the Colorado and other rivers. Water experts think that future wars will be fought over water, not over oil. Modern technologies hopefully will tap sun and wind for energy. Oil can be replaced by alternative fuels. Water cannot. Oil-rich countries are often water-poor, so that many religious and territorial conflicts are aggravated by a clash over water resources.

As a physician deeply involved in integrative medicine (using conventional as well as alternative methods), I cannot overstate the importance of water for health—that is why I wrote this book. Water has been used for medical purposes since prehistoric times. Now we need to rediscover the healing benefits of water long known to ancient cultures. This discovery might prompt more awareness of our worldwide water crisis.

Desert people have a huge reverence for water. They save every drop—whereas we don't mind letting the water run while we brush our teeth, taking our water wealth for granted. But people in the desert often suffer from premature kidney failure because of constant dehydration. We here are luckier—but with it comes responsibility.

Water is universally used in holy rituals of many world religions. Water is sacred. Honoring and protecting water will guarantee our well-being and health, and the health of future generations.

So I end this book with a plea to conserve Earth's water and other resources. We must all work together to preserve our most precious resource. It's not as daunting as you might think. There are so many simple steps we can take:

- Take shorter showers.
- Keep lawn sprinklers on every other day, not every day, and turn them off when you're expecting rain.
- Check for leaks in your home faucets on a regular basis.
- Be sure never to litter in water sources like rivers, lakes, and oceans.
- Don't let the tap run while you brush your teeth.
- Don't have a water-intensive garden in dry areas of the country.

- Dispose responsibly of toxic waste, and minimize activities that contribute to toxic waste.
- Drive a fuel-efficient car; doing so helps prevent the greenhouse effect, which depletes the earth of its water supply.
- Use an air conditioner only for the elderly, sick, and frail or in really high temperatures. Air conditioners waste precious energy (often gained by water power harvested with dams) and contribute to the greenhouse effect, too.

Don't live wastefully, and we'll all be able to benefit from an abundance of the most important life-giving resource on Earth: fresh, clean water.

SELECTED REFERENCES

Part 1

Ball, P. 2001. *Life's Matrix: A Biography of Water.* Los Angeles: University of California Press, Berkeley.

Marks, W. E. 2001. *The Holy Order of Water: Healing Earth's Waters and Ourselves.* Great Barrington, MA: Bell Pond Books.

Shiva, V. 2002. *Water Wars: Privatization, Pollution, and Profit* (winner of the Alternative Nobel Prize, 1993). Cambridge, MA: South End Press.

Part 2

Alexander, F. M. 1996. *The Use of Self.* London: Gollancz.

Douillard, J. 2001. *Body, Mind, and Sport.* New York: Three Rivers Press.

Feldenkrais, M. 1990. *Awareness Through Movement: Health Exercises for Personal Growth.* San Francisco: Harper Collins.

Scaravelli, V. 1991. *Awakening the Spine: The Stress-Free New Yoga That Works with the Body to Restore Health, Vitality, and Energy.* San Francisco: Harper Collins.

Todd, M. E. 1937. *The Thinking Body: A Study of the Balancing Forces of Dynamic Man.* New York: Dance Horizons, Inc.

Trager, M., with C. Hammond. 1995. *Movement as a Way to Agelessness: A Guide to Trager Mentastics.* Barrytown, NY: Station Hill Press.

Part 3

Colbin, A. 1986. *Food and Healing: How What You Eat Determines Your Health, Your Well-Being, and the Quality of Your Life.* New York: Ballantine Books.

Gibbons, E. 1962. *Stalking the Wild Asparagus.* New York: David McKay Company, Inc.

Hyman, M. 2006. *UltraMetabolism: The Simple Plan for Automatic Weight Loss.* New York: Scribner.

Pitchford, P. 1993. *Healing with Whole Foods: Oriental Tradition and Modern Nutrition.* Berkeley, CA: North Atlantic Books.

Pollan, M. 2006. *The Omnivore's Dilemma: A Natural History of Four Meals.* New York: Penguin Press.

Tiwari, M. 1995. *Ayurveda: A Life of Balance.* Rochester, VT: Healing Arts Press.

Part 4

Blumenthal, M., et al. 1998. *The Complete German Commission E Monographs.* Boston: American Botanical Council.

Duke, J. A. 1997. *The Green Pharmacy.* New York: St. Martin's Press.

Mitchell, W. 2003. *Plant Medicine in Practice: Using the Teachings of John Bastyr.* St. Louis: Churchill Livingstone.

Tyler, V. E. and S. Foster. 1993. *Honest Herbal: A Sensible Guide to the Use of Herbs and Related Remedies.* Binghamton, NY: Haworth Herbal Press.

Part 5

Csikszentmihalyi, M. 1990. *Flow: The Psychology of Optimal Experience.* New York: HarperPerennial.

Kabat-Zinn, J. 1994. *Wherever You Go, There You Are: Mindful Meditation in Everyday Life.* New York: Hyperion.

Moore, T. 1992. *Care of the Soul: A Guide for Cultivating Depth and Sacredness in Everyday Life.* New York: HarperPerennial.

Norris, K. 1993. *Dakota: A Spiritual Geography.* New York: Houghton Mifflin.

Sogyal, R. 1992. *The Tibetan Book of Living and Dying.* San Francisco: Harper Collins.

Wright, R. 1994. *The Moral Animal: Evolutionary Psychology and Everyday Life.* New York: Vintage Books.

General Reference

Engel, C. 2002. *Wild Health: How Animals Keep Themselves Well and What We Can Learn From Them.* New York: Houghton Mifflin.

Fleckenstein, A. and R. Weisman. 2006. *Healthy to 100: Aging with Vigor and Grace.* Deerfield Beach, FL: Health Communications, Inc.

Kneipp, S. 2003. *My Water Cure.* Whitefish, MT: Kessinger Publishing. (Orig. pub. 1886.)

Weil, A. 1995. *Spontaneous Healing.* New York: Fawcett Columbine.

Weisman, R., with B. Berman. 2003. *Own Your Health: Choosing the Best from Alternative and Conventional Medicine.* Deerfield Beach, FL: Health Communications, Inc.

INDEX

Aches
    cold showers for, 6
    herbs for, 32
Acne, healing treatment for, 47
Adaptogens, herbs as, 184
Addictions, food, being overweight
        and, 151
Asthenic people, 14
African violets, 18
Aging, herbs for, 32
Aglaonema, 18
Airola, Paavo, 131
Alaria, 172
Algae, as ocean herb, 172
Allergies, food, weight gain and,
        141–42
Allspice, 175
Almond oil, sweet, 32
Aloe vera, 182
Aluminum, 145
Alzheimer's, 145
American ginseng, 179, 184
Anger, herbs for, 32
Anti-inflammatory foods, 125–28
Anxiety
    herbs for, 32
    meditation for, 111

Apple cider vinegar, 32, 33
Apples, 198
Arnica cream, 32
Arthritis
    healing treatment for, 47
    herbs for, 32
Arugula, 175
Ashwaganda, 184
Asian ginseng, 184
Asthma
    dry brushing of skin for, 60–61
    healing treatment for, 55
Astragalus, 184
Athletic people, 14
Ayurvedic oil baths, 20–21

Bachelor's button flowers, 178
Back. *See also* Posture
    arching one's, 92–93
    lazy exercises for, 93–94
Back bends, for posture, 105–6
Bad cholesterol, cold-water therapy
        and, xii
Balance
    cold water for maintaining, 8–10
    exercises, 94
    importance of, 191–92

life, 185–87
maintaining, 7–8
Bamboo, for bathroom spas, 18
Barefoot walking, 55, 60–61
Basil, 175, 183
    holy, 184
Bath oils, for bathroom spas, 19
Bathrooms, converting, into spas,
    17–19
Baths
    cold massage, 34
    cold sitz, 33–34
    fever-reducing, 38–39
    foot, 35
    happy half, 33–34
    herbal, 31–33
    mud, 37–38
    saltwater, 36
    treatments for health conditions
        in, 29
    warm, 30–31
    warm-to-hot, 39–40
Bathtubs, healing treatments in,
    29–30
Bay leaf, 175
Beans, 121
Bear medicine, 180
Bingen, Hildegard von, 41
Binges, food, meditation for, 111–12
Birch leaves, 178
Black cohos, 182
Black pepper, 175, 183
Blackberry leaves, 178
Blood pressure. See also High blood
    pressure
    cold showers and, 5, 8, 9
    hot water and, 10
    meditation for, 111–12
Body constitutional types, categories
    of, 14
Body functions, water and, 4

Body temperature, 4
BodyLift device, 104–5
Bone health, herbs for, 183
Bone pain, herbs for, 32
Bones, broken, herbs for, 32
Borage, 175
Boredom
    being overweight and, 150
    meditation for, 111
Bran, 33
Breakfast tips, 129
Breast-feeding, herbs and, 171
Breathing, 107–8
    basics of, 108–9
    cold showers for, 5
    evening, 110
    exercises, 108–11
    meditation for, 111–12
    morning, 109–10
    yoga, 109
Breathing problems, healing
    treatment for, 47
Bronchitis, herbs for, 32
Broth, vegetable, recipe for, 144–45
Bruises, external, herbs for, 183
Brushing of skin, dry, 55, 60–61

Calcium
    dairy products and, 135–36
    herbs for, 183
Calendula petals, 32, 178
Camphor, 32
Cancer, cold showers and, 5
Candles, health risks of, 18
Capsules, herbal, 167
Cardamom, 175
Carnation flowers, 178
Carpal tunnel syndrome, healing
    treatment for, 41
Cayenne, 176
Celery seed, 183

Cellulite
    dry burshing of skin for,
        60–61
    healing treatment for, 55
Chamomile flowers, 32, 33, 58, 175,
        181, 183
Cherry blossoms, 178
Chervil, 183
Chest wrappings, 64–65
Chicory flowers and buds, 178
Chinese Pearl Cream, 56
Chives, 175, 176
Chlorella, 147–48
Chocolate, benefits of, 132
Cholesterol, bad, cold-water therapy
        and, xii
Chronic pain
    cold showers for, 5
    meditation for, 111
Cider vinegar, apple, 32, 33
Cilantro, 147, 175
Cinnamon, 176, 183
Circulation problems
    dry brushing of skin for, 60–61
    healing treatment for, 29, 47, 55
    herbs for, 32
Citrus blossoms (lemon, orange,
        grapefruit, etc.), 178
Clary, 32, 181
Cleansing, body, with herbs,
        147–48
Cloves, 176
Cocoa, benefits of, 132
Cold arm bath, 42
Cold eye wash, 45
Cold knee/leg gush, 35–36
Cold massage bath, 34
Cold mouth rinse, 42
Cold showers, 23–27
    alternating hot and, 27–28
    benefits of, 5–6

blood pressure and, 9
cold bodies and, 25
Cold sitz bath (happy half bath),
        33–34
Cold washes, 23
Cold water
    benefits of, 5–6
    for maintaining balance, 8–10
Cold-water therapy, xi
Cold-water treading, 47, 53–54
Cold-water treatments, rules for,
        12–15
Cold wrappings, 63–64
Colds, See Common cold
Colors, for bathroom spas, 17–18
Comfrey, 32, 171
Common cold
    herbs for, 32
    herbs to fight against, 180
    restoring balance and, 195–96
Compresses, alternating hot and cold,
        55, 62–63
Conditioners, for bathroom spas, 19
Congestion, herbs for, 32
Connection with nature and soil, 190
Constipation
    healing treatment for, 47, 55, 56
    herbs for, 32
    restoring balance and, 196–98
Cornflower, 178
Cravings, food, 153
Curry, 176

Dairy products, 134–35
    calcium and, 135–36
Dandelion, 147, 178, 183
Decade of Water, United Nations,
        3, 206
Depression
    being overweight and, 150
    meditation for, 111–12

Detoxification
    cold showers for, 5
    dry brushing of skin for, 60–61
    healing treatment for, 47
Diagonal stretch, 88–89
Diets
    nutrition and, 140
    Stone Age, 119–20
    weight loss, being overweight and,
        150
Dill, 175
Dill weed, 183
Dinner tips, 129–30
Dr. Alexa's Cough Tea, 180
Dr. Alexa's Stir-fry, 138
Dried foods, 121
Dried herbs, 166, *See also* Herbs
Dry brushing of skin, 55, 60–61
Duke, James, 160
Dulse, 172

Eating. *See* Meals
Eating habits, being overweight and,
    150
Echinacea flowers and leaves, 178, 180
Eczema, herbs for, 32
Edema, cold showers for, 6
Egg timer, 112
Eleuthero, 184
Enemas, 55
    herbal, 168
    warm-water, 65–66
Energy, lack of, healing treatment
    for, 29
English daisies whole plants, 178
Eucalyptus, 32, 58
European Natural Medicine (ENM)
    categories of body types in, 14
    food and, 116
Evening breathing, 110
Evening primrose, 32
Evergreens, 32

Exercise(s), *See also* Movement
    arching one's back, 92–93
    back, 93–94
    balance, 94
    diagonal stretch, 88–89
    excuses for, 78–85
    hanging out, 96–97
    heavy, 98
    isometric, 74
    lazy, 88–97
    light, 97
    medium, 97–98
    micro movements, 89–90
    micro movements in car, 91–92
    micro movements on floor, 90–91
    morning bed, 97
    movement and, 73–74
    for perfect posture, 102–3
    ski machine, 95
    tricks for starting, 77–78
    two-minute, 76
    weight lifting, 95–96
Exhaustion, herbs for, 32
Extracts, 167
Eyes, tired, healing treatment for, 41

Face masks, 55, 57
Facecloths, for bathroom spas, 19
Facial steam, 55, 58
Fasting, 142–47
    benefits of, 144
    guidelines for, 145–47
    preparing for one-day, 144–45
Fatigue
    cold showers for, 5
    healing treatment for, 29
    herbs for, 32
    meditation for, 111–12
Fats, hydrogenated, 152
Feet, tired, healing treatment for,
    29, 55
Feldenkrais Method, 83

Female pains, herbs for, 32
Feng shui, 59–60
Fennel, 175, 183
Fenugreek, 176, 183, 197, 198
Fermented foods, 121
Ferns, for bathroom spas, 18
Fever, healing treatment for, 30, 56
Feverfew flowers and leaves, 178
Fever-reducing baths, 38–39
Ficus benjamina, 18
Five Pillars of Health (Kneipp), ix
Five Water Essentials, x–xi
    human body and, xi
    reasons for needing, xi
    sample day with, 202–3
    sample week with, 203–4
    for weight loss program, 152–53
Five-minute meditation, 111–12
Flax seed, 197
Flexner, Abraham, 159
Flexner Report, 159
Flu, herbs for, 32
Food addictions, being overweight
    and, 151
Food allergies, weight gain and,
    141–42
Food binges, meditation for,
    111–12
Food cravings, 153
Food shopping, 148
Foods
    anti-inflammatory, 125–28
    considerations when choosing,
        117–18
    dried, 121
    fermented, 121
    fresh, organic, 121–25, 148
    freshness and, 115–117
    Freshness Pyramid for, 118–19
    healthful, soil and, 120
    inflammatory, 125–28
    phytonutrients in, 121–23

Stone Age diet and, 119–20
    wrong, 151
Footbaths, 35
    for head colds, 11
Forsythia flowers, 178
Fountains, indoor, 59–60
Foxglove, 171
Fresh herbs, 165–66. *See also* Herbs
Freshness Pyramid, for foods, 118–19
Fruits, 121

Garbanzos, 121
Gardening, water-preserving, 207
Garlic, 184, 197, 198
Ginger, 176, 184, 197, 198
Ginkgo, 179
Ginkgo biloba, 182
Ginseng, 179, 183
    American, 184
    Asian, 184
    Siberian, 184
Goldenrod flowers and upper leaves,
    178
Good King Henry, 178
Government diet recommendations,
    150
Grains, 121
Gratitude, for meals, 130
Green, meaning of, 156–58
Green Pharmacy, The (Duke), 160
Gums
    healing treatment for, 41
    herbs for, 182

Habits, eating, being overweight and,
    150
Hair
    cold showers for, 6
    herbs for, 32
Hanging out exercises, 96–97
Happy half bath (cold sitz bath),
    33–34

Hawthorn, 183
Hayflowers, 32
Head dunk, 44
Headaches, tension
  healing treatment for, 41, 47
  meditation for, 111–12
Headstands, 104–5
Healing treatments, 55–56. *See also*
  specific treatment
  in bathtub, 29–30
  at public establishments, 47
  at sinks, 41
Heart problems, herbs for, 183
Heaters, for bathroom spas, 18
Hebel, Johann Peter, 67–69
Hemorrhoids, cold showers for, 6
Herbal baths, 31–33
Herbal capsules, 167
Herbal enemas, 168
Herbal juices, 166
Herbal lotions, 168
Herbal ointments, 168
Herbal products, tips for choosing,
  168–70
Herbal suppositories, 168
Herbal syrups, 167
Herbal tablets, 167–68
Herbal tea, 172–73
  brewing, 177
  Dr. Alexa's cough tea, 180
  growing, 176–79
  for stress, memory, or anxiety,
    179
Herbal tea bags, 166
Herbal teas, herbs for, 178–79
Herbs, 155–56
  active ingredients in, 169
  for aromatherapy for sleep, 181
  body cleansing with, 147–48
  buying, 168–70
  for calcium and bone health, 183

for common cold, 180
correct dosages for, 170–71
dried, 166
fresh, 165–66
for gums, 182
healing tradition of, 158–63
interactions and, 171
investigating, 170
for kitchens, 175
medicinal, 160
menopausal, 181–82
ocean, 172
for organs, 183
pollution and, 171
as remedies, 161
safety guidelines for, 171
for sleep, 181
for specific conditions, in baths,
    32–33
standardized, 169–70
as tonics, 161, 184
types of, 165–68
for weight loss, 151
High blood pressure. *See also* Blood
    pressure
  healing treatment for, 41
  meditation for, 111–12
  restoring balance and, 198
Hippocrates, 158
Hijiki, 172
Hollyhock flowers, 178
Holy basil, 184
Home spas
  converting bathrooms into, 17–19
  essentials for, 19–21
Homeostasis, 7
Honeysuckle flowers, 178
Hops, 33, 179, 181
Horsetail, 32
Hot showers, alternating cold and,
    27–28

Hot tubs, 49
Human body
    effect of cold water on, 11
    effect of warm water on, 10–11
    Five Water Essentials and, xi
Hydrogenated fats, 152
Hypertension. *See* High blood
    pressure

Immune training, healing treatment
    for, 47
Indecisiveness, healing treatment
    for, 41
Indian root, 180
Indoor fountains, 55, 59–60
Infections, cold showers and, 5
Inflammatory foods, 125–28
Infusions, 166–67
Inhalations, 167
Insomnia
    cold showers for, 6
    healing treatment for, 55, 56
    herbs for, 33, 181
    meditation for, 111–12
    restoring balance and, 199–200
    wet socks treatment for, 60
Isometric exercises, 74

Jacuzzis, 49
Jade plant, 178
Jasmine, 32, 33
Johnny-jump-up flowers and leaves,
    178
Joint pain, healing treatment for, 29,
    55
Juices, avoiding, for weight loss,
    149
Juniper, 32

Kava kava, 179
Kegel exercises, 79

Kelp, 32, 33, 172
Kidney functions, cold showers
    for, 6
Kitchen herbs, 175
Kneipp, Sebastian, ix, 1, 5, 10, 12, 33,
    60, 137, 139, 163, 187
Kombu, 172
Kudzu flowers and leaves, 178

Lamb, organic, 123
Lavender, 32, 33
Laver, 172
Leg gush/cold knee, 35–36
Legs, tired, healing treatment for,
    29, 47
Legumes, 121
Lemon balm, 33, 175, 176, 179, 181
Lemon essential oil, 59
Lemon grass, 33
Lentils, 121
Licorice, 183, 184
Life balance, 185–87
Life energy (qi), 192–93
Lilac flowers, 178
Linden flower essential oil, 59
Linden flowers, 178
Liver problems, herbs for, 183
Loneliness, being overweight and,
    150
Lotions
    for bathroom spas, 19
    herbal, 168
Lung afflictions
    healing treatment for, 41
    meditation for, 111–12
Lymphatic circulation, cold showers
    for, 6

Maitake mushroom, 184
Marjoram, 32, 175, 183
Marshmallow flowers, 178

Masks, face, 57
Meals, guidelines for, 129–31
Media, being overweight and, 150
Medicinal herbs, 160
Meditation, 111–12
Menopausal herbs, 181–82
Menthol, 32, 33
Messenger molecules, 9
Metabolism
  cold showers and, 5
  hot water and, 10
Micro movements, 74, 89–90
  in car, 91–92
  on floor, 90–91
Milk, 134–35
  calcium and, 135–36
  soy, 136
Milk thistle, 147, 183
Mints, 176
Mirrors, for bathroom spas, 18
Miso, 121
Mood, cold showers and, 5
Morning bed exercises, 97
Morning breathing, 109–10
Motivation, cold showers and, 5
Movement, 67–70. *See also*
    Exercise(s)
  benefits of, 70–71
  getting started, 75–76
  tips for, 88
  two-minute exercises for, 76
  types of, 74
Mud baths, 37–38
Multiple sclerosis (MS), healing
    treatment for, 47
Muscle pain, healing treatment for,
    29, 55
Muscle spasms, herbs for, 32
Myrrh tincture, 182

Nasturtium flowers, buds, leaves,
    seedpods, 178
Natural spring water, 133
Neuro-immuno-endocrine system, 9
Nonalcoholic extracts, 167
Nori, 172
Nose, stuffy, healing treatment for,
    41
Nutmeg, 176
Nutrition, diet and, 140
Nuts, 121

Oak bark extract, 33
Oats, 33, 56
Obesity, 75, *See also* Overweight
Ocean herbs, 172
Ocean therapy (thalassotherapy), 36
Ointments, herbal, 168
Olive leave extract, 180
Olive oil, 20, 32, 33
  for lotions, 19
Orange essential oil, 32
Oregano, 175, 176, 183
Organic foods, 121–25, 148. *See also*
    Foods
Organic lamb, 123
Osha, 180
Overweight, common reasons for
    being, 149–52. *See also* Obesity

Pains
  cold showers for, 6
  herbs for, 32
  meditation for, 111
Palms, 18
Panic attacks, meditation for, 111
Pansy flowers and leaves, 178
Paprika, 176
Parsley, 175, 183

Passionflower, 179, 181
Pau d'arco, 180
Peas, 121
Pennyroyal, 171
Peperomia, 18
Pepper, black, 175, 183
Peppermint, 59, 175
Petunia flowers, 178
pH (acidity/alkalinity) balance, 4
Philodendrons, for bathroom spas, 18
Phytonutrients, foods high in,
    121–23
Pigweed, 183
Pilates, 83
Pine, 32
Plantain leaves, 178
Plants, for bathroom spas, 18
Pool gymnastics, 48
Poppy seed, 183
Posture, 99–100
    exercises for, 102–6
    health conditions that affect, 102
    tips for perfect, 100–102
Prana, 109
Pregnancy, herbs and, 171
Premenstrual syndrome (PMS),
    meditation for, 111–12
Prostate, herbs for, 183
Prunes, 197
Psycho-neuro-immune system, 9
Psyllium, 197
Purslane leaves, 178, 183
Pycnic people, 14

Qi (life energy), 192–93

Raspberry leaves, 178
Red clover, 175, 182, 183
Reishi mushrooms, 184

Remedies, herbs as, 161
Respiratory diseases, healing
    treatment for, 56
Rhodiola, 184
Rhythms, natural, importance of
    keeping with, 189–90
Roman baths, 53
Rose hips, 178
Rose petals and leaves, 178
Rose water, 56
Rosemary, 175, 176
Roses, 32, 33
Russian baths, 53

Sadness, being overweight and,
    150
Safety guidelines, for herbs, 171
Sage, 32, 175, 176, 180, 183
Saint-John's-wort, 179
Saltwater baths, 36
Saltwater nose rinse, 42–44
Sandalwood, 181
Sauerkraut, 121
Saunas, 47, 49–52
    timetable for, 51–52
Savory, 175, 183
Saw palmetto berries, 182
Schisandra, 184
Sciatica, herbs for, 32
Seaweeds, as ocean herb, 172, 183
Shampoos, for bathroom spas, 19
Showers
    alternating hot and cold, 27–28
    cold, 5–6, 23–27
Siberian ginseng, 184
Sinks
    cold arm bath, 42
    cold eye wash, 45
    cold mouth rinse, 42

head dunk, 44
saltwater nose rinse, 42–44
treatments for health conditions
    using, 41
Sinus problems, healing treatment
    for, 55
Sitz bath, cold, 33–34
Ski machine exercises, 95
Skin
    cold showers for, 5
    cold water on, 9
    dry, itchy, healing treatment for,
        29, 47
Skin care
    face masks for, 57
    facial steam for, 58
    with water, 56–58
Skin disease, warm herbal baths for,
    31
Skin inflammation, herbs for, 32
Skin problems
    healing treatment for, 55
    herbs for, 33
Skullcap, 179, 181
Sleep
    aromatherapy for, 181
    herbs for, 181
Sleeping pills, 199
Sleeplessness. See Insomnia
Snapdragon flowers, 178
Soap, 24, 56
Soil, healthy food and, 120
Solanine, 128
Sorrel leaves, 179
Soy milk, 136
Soybean oil, 32
Spas, See Home spas
Spathophyllum, 18
Spices, 175–76

Spirulina, 32
Sport injuries, healing treatment for,
    47
Standardized herbs, 169–70
Starches, avoiding, for weight loss,
    149
Steam baths, 47, 52–53
Steam inhalation, 55, 58–59
Stinging nettle, 147, 179, 183, 184
Stock, vegetable, recipe for, 144–45
Stomach problems, herbs for, 183
Stone Age diet, 119–20
Stone fruit blossoms, 178
Storm, Theodor, 205
Stress
    being overweight and, 150
    cold showers for, 6
    healing treatment for, 29, 47, 55
    herbs for, 33
    meditation for, 111–12
Stroke, healing treatment for, 47
Sugars, avoiding, for weight loss, 149
Supplements, 136–37
Suppositories, herbal, 168
Sweet almond oil, 32
Sweet violets, 198
Swelling, cold showers for, 6
Syndrome X, 139
Syrups, herbal, 167

Tablets, herbal, 167–68
Tai chi, 83
Tea, herbal, 172–73
Tea tree oil, 32, 59, 182
Teeth, healing treatment for, 41
Temperatures, water, 27
Tension headaches, healing treatment
    for, 41
Thalassotherapy (ocean therapy), 36

Thales, 3
Thyme, 32, 33, 175, 176, 183
Tinctures, 167
Tonics, herbs as, 161, 184
Touch, importance of, 190–91
Towels, for bathroom spas, 19
Toxicity, herbs for, 33
Trans-fatty acids, 152
Treading, cold-water, 53–54
Treatments, *See* Healing treatments
Turkish baths, 53
Turmeric, 176

United Nations Decade of Water, 3,
    206

Valerian, 33, 179, 181
Vanilla, 176
Vapor rub, 59
Vaporizers, 58–59
Varicose veins
    cold showers for, 6
    healing treatment for, 29, 47, 55
    herbs for, 32
Vegetable broth, recipe for,
    144–45
Vegetables, 121
Vinegar, apple cider, 32, 33
Violet flowers and leaves, 179
Violets, sweet, 198
Vitamins, 136–37

Walking barefoot, 55, 61–62
Walks, daily, importance of, 190
Warm baths, 30–31
Warm water, effect of, on human
    body, 10–11
Warm-to-hot baths, 39–40
Warm-water enemas, 65–66

Water
    benefits of cold, 5–6
    benefits of drinking, 132–33
    body functions and, 4
    conservation measures for,
        207–8
    consumption tips for, 133–34
    diminishing supplies of, 206
    drinking, before meals, for weight
        loss, 148
    functions of, inside human body,
        4–5
    humans and, 3–4
    natural spring, 133
    as political issue, 206–7
    temperatures for, 27
    UN Decade of Water, 3, 206
Water exercise, 47, 48
Water treatments, xii
Watercress, 175, 183
Weight gain
    being overweight and, 151
    food allergies and, 141–42
Weight lifting, slow motion, 95–96
Weight loss, 139–40
    avoiding sugars, starches, and
        juices for, 149
    cleansing with herbs and, 147–48
    drinking water before meals and,
        148
    fasting and, 142–47
    Five Water Essentials for,
        152–53
    food allergies and, 141–42
    food shopping and, 148
    herbs for, 151
    organic foods and, 148
Weight loss diets, being overweight
    and, 150

Wet socks against insomnia, 55, 60, 299
Whirlpools, 47, 48–49
Wild strawberry flowers and leaves, 179
Wild yam, 182
Wintergreen, 32
Witch hazel, 56
Worries, herbs for, 32
Wounds, herbs for, 183

Wrappings, 55
  chest, 64–65
  cold, 63–64
Wrong foods, being overweight and, 151

Yarrow, 33
Yoga, 83
Yoga breathing, 109
Yogurt, 33